Curves,
Twists
AND
Bends

of related interest

The Insightful Body
Healing with SomaCentric Dialoguing
Julie McKay
ISBN 978 1 84819-030-6

Yoga Therapy for Every Special Child
Meeting Needs in a Natural Setting
Nancy Williams
Illustrated by Leslie White
ISBN 978 1 84819 027 6

Qigong for Multiple Sclerosis
Finding Your Feet Again
Nigel Mills
ISBN 978 1 84819 019 1

Managing Stress with Qigong
Gordon Faulkner
Foreword by Carole Bridge
ISBN 978 1 84819 035 1

Body Intelligence
Creating a New Environment
2nd edition
Ged Sumner
ISBN 978 1 84819 026 9

Meet Your Body
CORE Bodywork and Rolfing Tools to Release Bodymindcore Trauma
Noah Karrasch
Illustrated by Lovella Lindsey
ISBN 978 1 84819 016 0

You Are How You Move
Experiential Chi Kung
Ged Sumner
ISBN 978 1 84819 014 6

Curves, Twists AND Bends

A Practical Guide to Pilates for Scoliosis

ANNETTE WELLINGS
with Alan Herdman

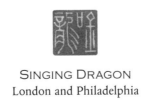

SINGING DRAGON
London and Philadelphia

First published in 2010
by Singing Dragon
116 Pentonville Road
London N1 9JB, UK
and
400 Market Street, Suite 400
Philadelphia, PA 19106, USA

www.singing-dragon.com

Library of Congress Cataloging in Publication Data
A CIP catalog record for this book is available from the Library of Congress

British Library Cataloguing in Publication Data
A CIP catalogue record for this book is available from the British Library

ISBN 978 1 84819 025 2

Printed and bound in Great Britain

In life, as in art, the beautiful moves in curves.

Edward George Earle Bulwer-Lytton (1803–1873)

Contents

Part 1   Understanding and Awareness

Part 2   Exercises for Flexibility and Posture

Part 3   Strategies for Living with Scoliosis

ACKNOWLEDGMENTS

This book is an accumulation of many years of exploring and discovering different facets of living with scoliosis. Annette Wellings would like to thank everyone who, throughout the years, has shared their views, insights, knowledge and time.

Special thanks to those individuals and their parents who shared their stories and experiences of scoliosis.

Thanks to Jane Mooney and Alan Herdman for being Annette's Pilates teachers; John Woodward, David Harrison and Julie Weaver for their insights and teaching; Dale Needham for computer assistance and manuscript preparation; Rosemary Rodwell for her constant support and encouragement; and to Paul for sharing the journey.

SAFETY NOTE

Introduction

The purpose of this book is to provide a practical guide to living with scoliosis. It includes ideas and strategies for coping with everyday living, as well as gentle exercises for flexibility, posture and muscle strength.

Scoliosis or 'lateral curvature of the spine' encompasses enormous variation. Each person's scoliosis is different. While we often hear of people who have 'got' scoliosis, there are striking differences between any two individuals diagnosed with curvature of the spine. In this way, scoliosis provides an opportunity for, and is a symbol of, individuality.

In the following pages, I describe the ideas, strategies and exercises that I have found effective in coping with my scoliosis in adulthood. It is important to note the purpose of the exercises in this book is to encourage flexibility and length, and enable the spine to be as healthy and supple as possible. The exercises are not designed to restructure the curve. They are suited for people with all types of scoliosis and can be modified according to the individual's specific needs.

I hope that this book provides you with a deeper understanding of options and ideas for exploring a way forward in living with scoliosis. Essentially, pick what suits you from these ideas. Choose the options and techniques that you find most effective for your particular scoliosis and lifestyle.

This book is divided into three parts. Part 1 focuses on understanding and awareness. It explains what scoliosis is, and describes physical and psychological aspects of spinal curvature. Part 2 describes exercises for flexibility, posture and muscle strengthening that are suitable for scoliosis. Part 3 outlines basic strategies and practical tips for coping with scoliosis in everyday life.

Understanding

AND

Awareness

WHAT IS SCOLIOSIS?

Scoliosis means lateral curvature and twisting of the spine. The spine curves from side to side, forming an S or C shape, rather than a straight line. The term 'scoliosis' comes from the Greek word 'skolios' meaning crooked, and 'skol' meaning 'twists and turns'.

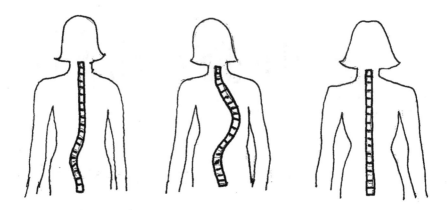

Spine with and without scoliosis

As the spine curves sideways, the individual vertebrae also twist and rotate, like the steps of a spiral staircase, around the vertical axis of the spinal column. That is, instead of each vertebra facing the same direction, there is a tendency to twist and rotate towards the direction of the curve. Because the ribs are attached to the vertebrae, this rotation of the vertebrae may create a 'hump' or prominence on one side of the back.

Structural and non-structural scoliosis

It is important to distinguish between structural and non-structural (functional) scoliosis. **Non-structural** scoliosis is less serious and tends not to alter the body structurally. This type of curve disappears when an X-ray is taken lying down or bending sideways. It can be caused by a variety of factors including muscle spasms, leg-length differences, injury, poor posture, or repeated unbalanced activity such as carrying heavy loads always on one side. Non-structural scoliosis tends to have only a small degree of curvature and therefore is usually much less noticeable. It is almost always reversible.

In contrast, **structural** scoliosis involves a spinal curvature that is always present. It is evident in X-rays taken lying on the back or bending sideways. An easy test for structural scoliosis is the forward-bending test. It involves bending forward at the waist, with the knees straight and head down, reaching the fingertips towards the floor. If the spine is straight or has only a non-structural curve, then both sides of the upper and lower back will be symmetrical and the hips will be level and even. If there is a structural scoliosis, then the rib cage and/or lower back will be asymmetrical. This unevenness may appear as a hump on one side of the torso. This basic test is part of the screening examination often used in schools to help identify scoliosis.

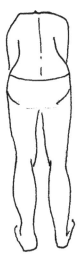 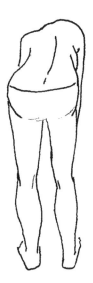

The forward-bending test

Symptoms

Scoliosis can often go unnoticed in its early stages as it is rarely painful in its formative years. It may be detected by symptoms such as:

- One shoulder appears higher than the other.

- One shoulder blade protrudes or sits out from the back.

- The waist is uneven – straight on one side and curved in on the other. You may see a crease at the waist on the curved side.

- A tendency to lean to one side. Rather than a straight vertical line from the head to the tailbone, the head seems shifted off to one side.

- One hip seems higher than the other.

- A rib 'hump' on one side of the back.

- A bulge on one side of the mid or lower back.

For those interested in a more technical description, here is a list of characteristics that may occur with scoliosis. Note that these vary depending on the individual case, the type and the severity of the curve.

- Imbalance in the paraspinal muscles, which run parallel to the spine. The muscles on the concave side of the curve appear weak and sunken, while the convex side (which the curve leans towards, i.e. the outside of the curve) tends to have a block of strong, well-developed muscle, forming a bulge effect.

- This muscle imbalance causes further distortion of the spinal column and uneven weight distribution over the facet joints. Some facet joints may become damaged by chronically working under increased pressure.

- Wedging of the vertebrae and discs. Due to the structure of the curve, vertebrae and discs become compressed and wedged on one side.

- Vertebral rotation. Vertebrae of the curve tend to rotate around the vertical axis of the spinal column, and become fixed in this rotated position.

- Rib prominence or 'hump'.

- Protrusion of one hip.

- 'Frozen chest' – limited chest expansion, respiratory dysfunction.

- Torso asymmetry – the thorax is skewed and off-centre or the pelvis is twisted and misaligned.

- Flat back syndrome.

- Kyphosis – a posture whereby the spine bends or arches forwards to an excessive degree (often creating rounded shoulders).

- Lordosis – a posture whereby the spine arches excessively backwards (often creating a 'swayback' effect).

- Decreased spinal mobility. Loss of flexibility in one or more segments of the curvature.

- Stenosis – abnormal narrowing of the spinal canal.

- Bone spurs.

- Arthritis.

- Gait and torso imbalance.

Idiopathic scoliosis

The majority of scoliosis cases are classed as 'idiopathic' which simply means that the cause is unknown. About 80–90 per cent of scoliosis cases fall into this idiopathic category.

While it is difficult to estimate precisely, about 20 in every 1000 youngsters will develop a lateral curvature. Out of these 20 cases, 15 will have only very slight curvatures of less than 20 degrees. Such mild cases usually do not require medical intervention, bracing or surgery. The remaining 5 of every 1000 will have curves greater than 20 degrees, but only one or two of these cases will require treatment (Schommer 2002).

Idiopathic scoliosis is divided into four categories based on the age at which the scoliosis develops:

- infantile: children under 3 years old

- juvenile: 3–9 years old

- adolescent: 10–18 years old

- adult: after skeletal maturity.

Adolescent idiopathic scoliosis, which develops around the onset of puberty, is by far the most common. It represents approximately 80 per cent of idiopathic scoliosis cases, and is much more frequent in girls than in boys. It usually becomes evident in girls between the ages of 10 and 14 years, and in boys between 12 and 15 years.

Causes

For those cases of scoliosis which are not idiopathic, this section briefly outlines some of the commonly recognized causes of curvature of the spine. They include congenital, neuromuscular, and degenerative factors.

Congenital scoliosis is caused by inborn spinal defects such as missing or fused vertebrae. ('Congenital' simply means a condition you were born with.) It usually becomes apparent at the age of two years or in children aged 8–13, as the spine grows more quickly, putting extra strain on the abnormal vertebrae.

Neuromuscular scoliosis may result from causes including:

- spinal cord injuries (paraplegia, quadraplegia)

- infectious diseases such as polio and tuberculosis

- cerebral palsy

- traumatic injury to the brain or spinal column

- muscular dystrophy

- neurological or muscle disorders.

Degenerative scoliosis usually occurs in older adults. It is caused by changes in the spine due to degeneration and arthritis. Abnormal bone spurs combined with weakening of ligaments and soft tissues of the spine can lead to spinal curvature.

Various conditions that affect bones and muscles linked with the spinal column may also result in scoliosis. These include:

- tumours, either benign or malignant

- spinal infections

- stress fractures and hormonal abnormalities that affect bone growth

- trauma caused by radiation, injury, burns or spasm.

Other factors that can cause scoliosis include leg-length inequality and diseases such as Marfan syndrome, rheumatoid arthritis, spina bifida and spinal muscular atrophy.

These are just some of the causes of scoliosis. As Hawes (2003, p.22) notes: 'Scoliosis is known to occur in response to numerous genetic, environmental and metabolic insults, but it may take years after the triggering event happens before the symptoms…actually show up. By then, it is impossible to go back and identify the specific cause in any given patient'. For readers wishing a detailed discussion of the complex variety of causes, *Scoliosis and the Human Spine* (Hawes 2003; see pp.12–22) would be a good starting point.

WIDE VARIATION OF TYPES

There is enormous variation in scoliosis cases. Scoliosis can include any or all of the vertebrae of the spine and exhibit a range of shapes. The form of each person's scoliosis varies according to:

- the location of the curve

- the size or magnitude of the curve

- the overall shape of the curve(s)

- the degree of vertebral rotation and rib hump

- the occurrence of front-to-back curves – kyphosis, lordosis and flat back.

Location of the curve

The vertebrae of the spine are divided into three groups. The bones of the neck are called **cervical** vertebrae, those in the upper back down to the waist are called **thoracic**, and the lower back vertebrae are named **lumbar**. The individual vertebrae are often called thus:

- the five lumbar vertebrae: L1–L5

- the 12 thoracic vertebrae: T1–T12

- the seven cervical vertebrae: C1–C7.

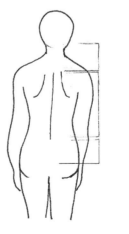 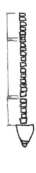

Cervical, thoracic and lumbar spine

Scoliosis is often classified according to the location of the curve. A 'lumbar' curve occurs in the five vertebrae of the lower back between the waist and the sacrum. A 'thoracic' curve occurs in the 12 thoracic vertebrae which are connected to the ribs. 'Cervical' scoliosis occurs in the seven top vertebrae below the skull. 'Thoracolumbar' scoliosis affects the vertebrae in both thoracic and lumbar sections of the spine.

Shape of the curve

Curvatures are often simplistically referred to as 'S' or 'C' shape. A C-shape curve leans to one side of the spinal axis, either right or left. An S-shape scoliosis curves to one side and then to the other, like two C-shape curves, one on top of the other, with one leaning left and the other leaning right.

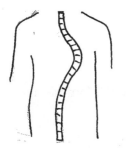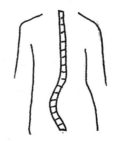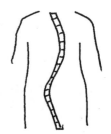

S- and C-shape curves

The shape of the curvature is often much more complex. The wide variety of scoliosis curves is illustrated in the figure on the next page.

Degree of the curve

Scoliosis is measured by the Cobb angle which grades the severity of the curvature by degree. A curve of less than 10 degrees is considered 'normal' and occurs commonly in healthy spines. Scoliotic curves are generally classified as mild (10–24 degrees), moderate (25–50 degrees), or severe (50 degrees or more).

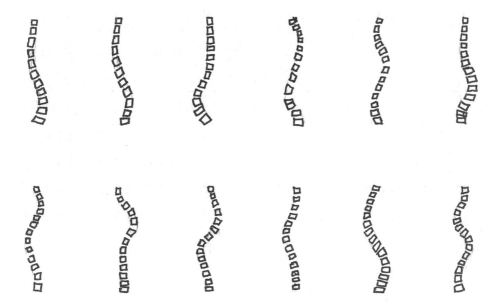

Some different shapes of curvature

To measure the Cobb angle, a line is drawn across the top and bottom vertebrae of the curve. Because the vertebrae in the curved spine are tilted, the two drawn lines intersect. The angle at the intersection of the two lines is the measurement of the magnitude of the curve. The more severe the curve, the more the vertebrae are tilted, and the greater the angle at the intersection of the drawn lines. A straight spine with no curves (and thus no tilting vertebrae) measures 0 degrees, as the two parallel lines do not intersect.

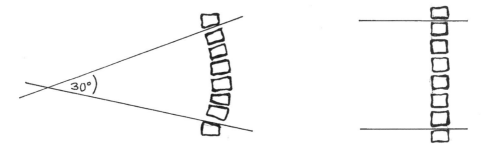

Cobb angle measurement of the spine

Vertebral rotation and rib hump

As the spine curves sideways, the vertebrae may also twist or rotate around the spinal axis. The degree of rotation is classified from Grade 0 – no rotation, Grade 1 – least severe, to Grade 4 – most severe. Vertebral rotation is usually measured from an X-ray or Magnetic Resonance Imaging (MRI) scan.

As a result of the rotated vertebrae, the rib cage (which is attached to the thoracic vertebrae) becomes twisted and pushed out of alignment. This shows up as a rib hump on one side of the upper back. The size of the rib hump often reflects the severity of the scoliosis. Usually the rib hump becomes more apparent in adult scoliosis. (The severity of a rib hump is measured by a 'scoliometer'.)

Kyphosis, lordosis and flat back

As well as curving sideways, the scoliotic spine can develop pronounced front-to-back or 'sagittal' curves. **Kyphosis** means that the spine bends forward. This pronounced forward bending in the upper back creates a hunching effect of the shoulders and upper body. **Lordosis** refers

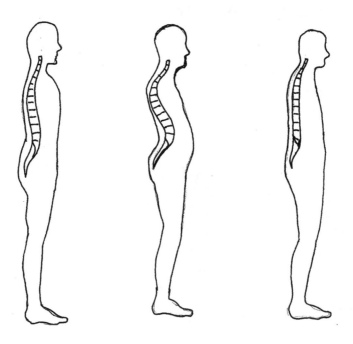

Normal (left), kyphosis and lordosis (centre), flat back (right)

Information chart for your scoliosis

Location of curve(s):

Cervical

Thoracic

Lumbar

Thoracolumbar

Degree of curve(s):

Vertebral rotation (shown as a protrusion on one side of the spine):

Lower back

Upper back

Rib hump

Front-to-back curve(s):

Kyphosis

Lordosis

Flat back

Overall shape of spine:

Mark out the shape of your curvature on the figure to the right.

C1

C7
T1

T12
L1

L5

to the spine arching backwards, causing the stomach and bottom to stick out. **Flat back** occurs when the spine actually becomes too flat, and loses its natural front-to-back sagittal curves. Flat back is present when the sagittal curve is less than 25 degrees.

Kyphosis, lordosis and flat back are common in scoliosis. All, some or none may occur in an individual case.

This variation in scoliosis cases highlights the importance of viewing the spine as a whole three-dimensional unit, like a helix that curves side to side, front to back, with twisting and rotation of the vertebrae within the spinal column.

Each scoliosis case is unique, according to the particular constellation of variable features discussed above. In living and coping effectively with scoliosis, it is important to be aware of and understand the features of your particular curvature.

In order to gain an overview and understanding of your particular case, the chart on page 23 is for you to fill in, as you gather information and awareness of the features of your individual curvature. It's a good idea to read all of this chapter before doing your chart. (Your medical practitioner should be able to help you confirm these data, if your case is under medical supervision.)

FOUR COMMON PATTERNS OF CURVATURE

While there is much variation in the shape of each scoliosis, four common patterns of curvature have been identified (Schommer 2002) and are commonly referred to:

1. **Right thoracic curve** occurs in the mid-back area. Usually the curve begins between the shoulder blades (around vertebrae T4–T6), and ends around the waist (at T11, T12 or L1). Note that approximately 90 per cent of thoracic curves lean to the right side. This curve pattern is often linked with a rib hump on the right side of the back.

2. **Lumbar curve** occurs in the lower back. It affects vertebrae from the waist region (T11 or T12) down to L5. Most cases (65–70%) of lumbar scoliosis lean to the left side. A lumbar curve will twist the pelvic girdle, creating the impression of uneven hips, with one hip higher and/or pushed further forward than the other.

3. **Thoracolumbar curve** creates a C-shape curve which usually begins between the shoulder blades (around T4–T6), and ends in the lower back (L3–L5). About 80 per cent of thoracolumbar curves lean to the right side. A thoracolumbar curve usually creates an asymmetrical torso, involving a rib hump and uneven waist and hips.

4. **Double or S-shape curve** is a combination of two curves: the upper curve is in the thoracic or chest area; the equal lower curve is in the lumbar spine. The lower curve leans in the opposite direction to the upper curve, providing a counterbalance. For S-shape scoliosis, the upper curve goes to the right side in 90 per cent of cases.

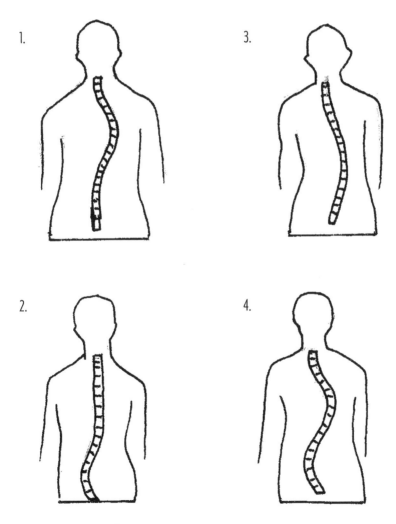

Four common patterns of curvature

The curve patterns illustrated on p.25 are prototypes which are commonly used in diagnosing and describing scoliosis. It is important to realize that these patterns are only rough maps. Not all scoliosis cases fall into these categories (e.g. cervical and thoracocervical curvatures affecting the neck area). Moreover, there is much variation and deviation of individual cases within each category. Smaller compensatory curves often occur above or below the major curve. Thus, the overall spinal profile may show three or four curves, due to smaller compensatory curves above and below the major curve.

Note: There are different systems for classifying scoliosis. For example, the Schroth method uses a distinct and different approach (see Lehnert-Schroth 2007).

THE PSYCHOLOGY OF SCOLIOSIS

While scoliosis is often viewed and treated as being a solely physical condition, it is also linked with levels of psychological distress. It is not uncommon for individuals with scoliosis to suffer emotionally and mentally as a consequence of having a cosmetic 'deformity' (Hawes 2003). In this section, we will look at common perceptions and coping mechanisms for how individuals deal with and perceive their scoliosis.

When first diagnosed with scoliosis, many individuals feel bewildered and embarrassed at being told that they have a physical 'deformity'. Feelings of being marked as different to friends, peers and other 'normal' people abound. This is compounded by a sense of helplessness and frustration of not knowing what to do.

A case study of adolescent scoliosis

When I was 13 my mother noticed that the skirt of my school uniform was always crooked and longer on one side. We went to a local doctor and then an orthopaedic surgeon who sat me down and explained that I had a major deformity that would be a constant and serious disability through life. I was told that the only sensible option was to weld the spine from neck to sacrum. The alternative was a wheelchair within decades.

I fled in tears, wishing that the consultant, his opinion and my twisted spine didn't exist. Life became more complicated and uneasy when I was nicknamed 'deformity' at school. In short, I felt ugly and deformed, ashamed of my body, confused and helpless about what to do.

There are different coping mechanisms in dealing with scoliosis:

Create an 'outer shell' of being normal, and ignore the scoliosis

In this way of coping, much focus and energy is put into appearing 'normal' to the outside world. For example, we create ways of dressing and moving so that the curvature and crookedness of the body is hidden or less obvious. We avoid situations where people can see our backs and bodies, such as swimming.

This shell of normality that we construct around ourselves enables us to 'get on with life' and function as normally as possible in the world around us. The flipside of this approach is that we ignore the scoliosis, until it becomes problematic with pain or progression of the curve.

In short, we create a protective shell or appearance of normality to the outside world, putting much emotional and physical energy into this protective cloak. Consequently, we tend to ignore and not to address the curvature and emotional issues that lie underneath.

Passive victim mode

Due to feelings of helplessness and lack of control, a passive victim perspective is easily adopted. We feel victimized and experience self-pity at the idea of having a spinal 'deformity' and 'degenerating' spinal curve. We become resigned to a downward spiral of helplessness and suffering. In this frame of mind, we often have limited knowledge and understanding of our individual scoliosis. Rather than explore options, we feel overwhelmed and leave the decisions and knowledge regarding the scoliosis to the professional authorities and experts.

In short, we resign ourselves to the belief that we are helpless and locked into an irreversible degeneration process in which our spines become increasingly rigid and distorted.

Determination and trying hard

At the other extreme to the 'passive victim' is the 'determined, try hard' mode. Individuals using this coping mechanism readily acknowledge that they have scoliosis. They become determined and try incredibly hard to succeed in dealing with their condition. This drive and determination extends into everyday behaviour, with a desire to 'pack a lot into life', 'live life to the full' and achieve success.

This determination as a coping strategy often translates in physical activity or physical therapy sessions as trying too hard, gripping and bracing. People in this mode often perceive the trait of determination and trying hard as vital to surviving and coping with scoliosis. In effect, trying hard and determination is seen as a way of keeping some control of the body. There is often a fear that without such determination, the curvature might increase or collapse.

An individual may consistently use one of these coping mechanisms, or may switch from one to another according to their particular circumstances. A constellation off all three may be used in different situations. These coping mechanisms can easily become a vicious cycle in which the individual is locked, experiencing great amounts of physical and emotional stress in trying to come to terms with their scoliosis.

It is important simply to be aware of which coping mechanisms we use in our own particular circumstances. From this awareness, a way out of this triad of coping mechanisms involves the following steps:

1. **Accept** that you've got scoliosis.

    ○ Recognize that it makes you unique, an individual.

    ○ Be observant of what you are experiencing physically and mentally.

    ○ Try not to judge your feelings. Try simply to observe.

2. **Get information:**

    ○ about your curvature (e.g. location, type and size of the curve)

    ○ about options available.

3. **Work out a way forward.**

    ○ Find the strategies and techniques that best suit you.

    ○ Look at all of the options, and make informed decisions.

THE MIND AND BODY LINK

In the 1600s, philosopher Rene Descartes proposed the idea that the mind and body are separate (otherwise called 'mind–body dualism'). His theory was hugely influential and still permeates the way many of us in the West think about ourselves. We are often socialized and educated to perceive the mind and the body as quite unrelated entities. In contrast, the notion of vital and complex links between mind and body is fundamental to Eastern philosophy and medicine. This view that there are profound linkages to be explored between the mind and body has gained some currency in the West in recent decades.

With scoliosis, it is a common perception that the body is a rigid, mechanical, deformed structure that becomes more distorted and twisted with age. The mind is regarded as separate to the body, operating on an intangible, unrelated level. This notion of separateness encourages the belief that the body is a distorted degenerating frame over which we have little control. For many people with scoliosis, attention is often focused on non-physical activity and refining the mind, as a way of compensating for the physical deformity.

The bossy muscle

With scoliosis, the torso appears uneven. There often develops a bulge or a hump on one side of the spine, opposite the curve. This hump or bulge forms a dominant muscle block. This muscle block is well developed and stands out in comparison to the weaker less-developed area on the opposite side of the spine.

The bossy muscle block tends to be strong, tight and overworked. It will dominate and kick in to do many physical movements, leaving the quieter muscle group on the other side of the spine weak and relatively unused or undeveloped.

In many everyday activities and during exercise, there is a tendency for the dominant muscles to do all of the work. This reinforces the asymmetry, with the bossy muscle group becoming even stronger and more dominant, and the sunken underemployed muscle group becoming weaker and un-confident with lack of use.

In observing my own scoliosis, I noticed a correlation or link between physical curvature and mind patterns. Specifically, the bossy muscle group kicked in and became more dominant and stronger when my mindset was focused on doing, trying hard, determination, and also in situations of stress. The physical symptoms of bracing my mind include:

- The bossy muscle group kicks in and does all of the work.

- The weaker side of the torso sinks further into the curve.

- The spine shortens and the helix shape of the spine increases (as if going into a protective shell).

- The rib cage rotates more, and the bossy muscle block feels tight and uncomfortable, as if it is actually pulling and rotating the rib hump further.

This was a revelation for me. For 40 years I had believed that my strength of mind and determination would compensate for, and possible even arrest, my spinal curvature. I was strongly proud of my willpower, for that seemed to balance my 'deformity'. I then realized that bracing myself with such steely determination and trying so hard was actually contributing to the physical asymmetry, making it worse.

I discovered that there was less pain and less physical distortion and gripping when I accepted the fact that my spine was twisted, and simply observed and stayed attuned to it, rather than bracing against it.

The spine bends under pressure

The helix shape of a spine with scoliosis tends to buckle physically under pressure, be this pressure physical or psychological. Physical pressures include:

- carrying heavy weights or loads

- strong weight-bearing or heavy spring-resistance exercise

- extreme physical tiredness through overexertion or lack of sleep

- extreme fatigue, such as through jetlag

- gripping, tensing and bracing the body, such as when trying too hard in physical exercise and activity

- maintaining a fixed sitting or standing posture, without moving, for long periods of time.

Psychological pressures include:

- stressful social and emotional situations

- mindsets of bracing, trying too hard, and straining to achieve.

Observing my own scoliosis, I found the degree of rib rotation and consequent size of the rib hump and the dominant muscle block increased markedly with emotional trauma (e.g. deaths of loved ones, radical shifts in personal circumstances). Similarly, extreme fatigue through jetlag, lack of sleep or excessive physical exertion triggered a noticeable increase in the size of the bossy muscle and the asymmetry of my torso.

The good news is that I found it possible to reverse these physical changes that were triggered by such pressure. Different exercises, techniques and strategies are discussed in the following sections of the book.

It is crucial therefore that, in exploring ways of living with scoliosis, we are aware of the physical and mental pressures that may have an impact on the curvature.

In terms of mindset, this means 'letting go' of the tendency to brace, control and try hard. This means instead: *accepting* the fact of the scoliosis; *observing* the physical and psychological way that you feel with it; and *exploring* ways of dealing with it (rather than bracing against it). In other words, shift your mind from control, forcing, gripping and bracing to accepting, observing, and exploring with curiosity.

In terms of the physical pressures impacting on the spine, it is vital that physical exercise programmes for scoliosis involve:

- lengthening and increasing flexibility of the spine

- teaching the bossy muscle block to 'let go' and switch off

- developing and strengthening the weak sunken side

- realigning the body

- avoiding high-impact and heavy weight-bearing exercise.

In the following section of this book, we will explore in detail some physical exercises for scoliosis.

PART 2

Exercises

FOR

Flexibility

AND

Posture

INTRODUCTION

In this section, we look at gentle exercises for improving flexibility and posture. The purpose of these exercises is to encourage suppleness and flexibility of the spine (rather than restructuring the curvature). If you want an exercise programme focusing on the structure of your specific curvature, it is vital to find a physical therapist with knowledge of scoliosis, who can tailor-make an individual programme according to your particular needs. Physical therapists specializing in the Katherina Schroth technique are trained to devise individual programmes for realigning spinal curvatures. In addition, various professional therapists specialize in yoga for scoliosis and rehabilitation Pilates.

The gentle flexibility exercises for scoliosis in this book draw on a number of approaches including rehabilitation Pilates, the Schroth method, Alexander technique and yoga. By doing ten minutes each morning and night, I have found these exercises to be an effective way of keeping my spine flexible, lengthened and relatively pain-free.

PRINCIPLES OF EXERCISES FOR SCOLIOSIS

The exercises in this book are based on the following principles:

Lengthening and flexibility of the spine

With scoliosis, the spine can become quite rigid and compressed, particularly in the areas of the curve. Lengthening and flexibility enable a more supple and healthy spine, and reduce pressure on compressed vertebral joints.

De-rotation of the spine, ribs and pelvis

In many cases of scoliosis, the lateral or sideways curve of the spine is accompanied by the rotation of vertebrae. It is vital to include some gentle de-rotation in an exercise programme, in order to mobilize the facet joints and vertebrae, and to counteract any tendency for the spine to rotate further.

Teaching the bossy dominant muscles to let go

With scoliosis, the muscles are strong, tight and well developed on one side of the spine, but weak and sunken on the other. There is a strong tendency for the bossy muscle block to do all of the work in many activities, movements and exercises. This reinforces the asymmetry and results in the bossy muscle group becoming even stronger and more dominant, while the weak side becomes less used and more sunken.

It is therefore important to teach the dominant muscle block to switch off and let go. Focus is on stretching out muscles that have become tight and overworked, and releasing them.

Teaching the weak side how to talk

The other side of the coin is to strengthen and lengthen the weak underdeveloped muscles. These muscles have become weak and unconfident through patterns of asymmetrical muscle use, because the dominant overused muscles tend to do all of the work. In effect we need to 'rewire the body', to encourage the pathways of muscle connection and energy flow on the weaker underdeveloped side of the torso.

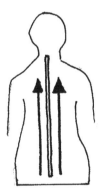 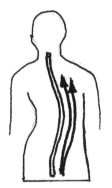 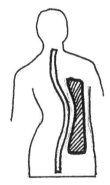

Patterns of energy flow and muscle connection

Pelvic stability

The pelvis provides the foundation for the spinal column. It is vital that the pelvis is aligned and stable, in order to provide the spine with a steady, balanced platform.

The pelvis may be likened to a basin, or the hull of a sailing boat which provides the base for the mast (in the same way that the pelvis provides the platform for the spine). Correct alignment is essential. The mast will tip forwards, sideways or backwards if the hull of the boat is off-kilter or misaligned.

The hull of the boat must also be stable and in good working condition, in order to support the mast. In the same way, it is important to tone and strengthen the muscles of the pelvic girdle, so that the pelvis is aligned and stable.

POSTURE AND ALIGNMENT

Before and during each exercise, it is important to have correct and balanced alignment. Before starting an exercise movement, spend a minute or two checking how the body is positioned, and realign your body towards a more symmetrical posture, if necessary. Checking alignment and keeping this awareness throughout the movement is an essential part of the exercise. It is not an optional bit that we can skip to save time! Doing an exercise without alignment runs the risk of actually reinforcing and increasing the imbalance of muscles and posture. If possible, work with a partner at first to ensure that your alignment is correct.

Here are the vital points to check for correct alignment:

Centreline

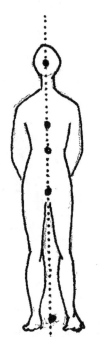

Centreline alignment

Make sure that there is a straight vertical line from your nose down to your feet, with all of these points in line:

- nose

- breast bone

- navel

- pubic bone

- central point between the feet.

Shoulders and hips

Make sure that your shoulders and hips are level, like two parallel horizontal lines.

Check also that each side of your torso is equal. That is, check that there is equal distance on each side between the lower rib and the hip. Often with scoliosis, the rib–hip distance is shorter on one side, due to one hip being higher or the rib cage sinking down on one side.

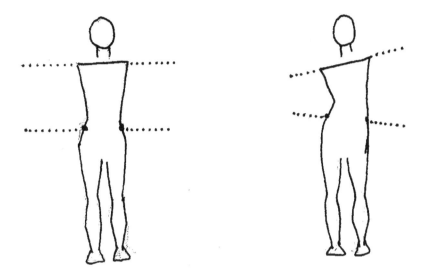

Alignment of the shoulders and hips

Pelvic alignment

Make sure that the pelvis is as balanced and aligned as possible. With scoliosis, there's a tendency for the pelvis to be off-balance. It's useful to check the following tendencies in your everyday posture and exercises, and gently correct them. (Stand in front of a full-length mirror or ask a friend to help you observe.)

- Check that your pelvis is not tilted excessively forward or backward. To check this, stand side-on to the mirror. An over-arched lower back happens when the pelvis is tilted forward. A flat lower back happens when the pelvis is tilted backward. If you notice this tendency, gently realign your pelvis to neutral position.

- Observing the body front-on, check if the pelvis is pushed across to one side, to the right or left (rather than centred in line with the head and navel).

- Check if one hip is higher than the other.

- Check if one hip is pushed further to the front than the other.

It may be useful to think of your pelvis as a basin which you constantly observe to detect any tendency to off-balance. Gentle correction back to neutral position will help re-pattern towards a more balanced alignment.

Weight distribution

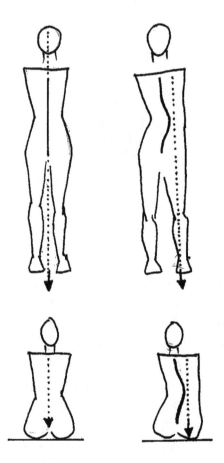

Equal weight distribution

Next, check that your weight is distributed evenly down the centreline of the body. If standing, check that the weight falls equally on both feet. If you are sitting, imagine equal weight on each buttock, or sit bone.

Be aware that, with scoliosis, weight distribution is often pushed to one side. We tend to lean towards and favour the dominant side which carries the weight.

To shift the weight back to the centreline of the body, imagine a golden beam of light, or alternatively a plumb-line, forming a vertical axis down the centreline of your body. Focus the weight to fall down this central vertical axis.

Length

Lengthen the neck and the spine, as if growing towards the ceiling. With scoliosis, we tend to collapse down into the curvature, and the spine sinks, compresses and shortens. In order to counteract this tendency, it is important to think of the head floating and the spine lengthening upwards.

Here are some useful images:

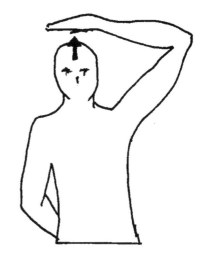

- Imagine a plant whose stem is constantly lengthening, growing towards the sun.

- Imagine a stream of energy flowing upwards through your spine and head, like toothpaste being squeezed out of a tube.

Lengthening technique

Another technique for getting the feel of lengthening is to place the flat palm of your hand a few centimetres above your head. Now lengthen your spine and 'grow' your head upwards towards your hand, trying to touch it. You'll notice that, with practice, you actually do lengthen and assume a taller posture with this exercise! (See exercise 19a for more details.)

INTRODUCING THE EXERCISES

Preparation

There are three golden rules for exercise preparation:

1. Check your alignment.

2. Let go of any tendency to brace physically or try too hard. Relax and enjoy the exercise movements. Observe and listen to how your body feels.

3. Now, lengthen the spine and float the head. Breathe into the sunken side to prepare (see exercise 25). Begin the movement, and breathe naturally throughout.

Before you begin an exercise, it's a good idea to read through the whole of the exercise, in order to get a sense of the overall movement. If you experience any pain doing an exercise, work within a smaller range and make the movement slower and gentler. If the discomfort persists, don't do that exercise, and check with your doctor or physical therapist.

The basic top ten exercises

Exercises 1–10

These are basic gentle exercises to keep the spine flexible and long. By doing five or ten minutes each morning and night, your back is encouraged to stay flexible. I usually do these exercises just before going to bed at night, and straight after rising each morning. This stretches out the body making it supple and prepared for the day ahead, and helps release stiffness and tension before sleeping each night.

This capsule of exercises can be done wherever you are. No props or equipment are required. All you need is:

- loose comfortable clothes (e.g. T-shirt or pyjamas!)

- a floor with carpet or a mat that's comfortable to lie on

- enough space to lie down with your arms and legs fully extended.

For the lying-down exercises, it is often useful to lie on a mat of flat foam, about 2–3 cm thick. This eases discomfort and relaxes tension in the back.

Work through the ten exercises and finish by repeating number 1, 'Reach for the sky'. If time or space does not permit on some days, simply modify your programme by selecting a few of the exercises. It's important to keep the spine mobile by doing these exercises regularly. Remember – a small amount on a regular daily basis is much more effective than a long session done every now and then, or whenever the pain gets bad.

Stretches

Exercises 11–15
Stretching is important for easing tightness, compression and imbalance in joints and muscles of the body.

De-rotation exercises

Exercises 16–18
With scoliosis, as the spine curves sideways, the vertebrae also rotate, like the steps in a spiral staircase. Gentle de-rotation exercises help mobilize the facet joints and vertebrae, and counteract any tendency for the spine to rotate further. The vital point to remember for de-rotation exercises is to keep a lengthened spine. Avoid any tendency to sink down into the curve, as you make the sideways movement.

Lengthening exercises

Exercises 1, 3, 19–22
Lengthening is vital, not only in exercise sessions, but also in everyday movement. It counteracts any tendency to shorten and compress the spine, or to sink down into the curve. Elongation helps relieve pressure on compressed vertebral joints. This is particularly important with vertebral wedging – when the vertebrae are wedged close together on one side of the curve.

Exercises for letting go of the bossy muscle

Exercises 13, 21–24
Our challenge with scoliosis is to allow the dominant muscle block to let go, so that it doesn't take over the role of other weaker muscles, and do all

of the work. Three ways of physically releasing the dominant muscles are: pressure and massage; stretching; and relaxation.

Exercises for teaching the weak side to talk

Exercises 14, 20, 25–29

Because of the dominance of the bossy muscle group, the muscles on the underdeveloped sunken side of the torso become weak and unconfident. To address this imbalance, we need to encourage pathways of muscle connection, energy flow, and strength in the weaker side. There are a variety of techniques including: breathing; touch stimulus; muscle strengthening; stretching and lengthening.

Exercises for pelvic stability

Exercises 30–34

The pelvis provides the foundation for the spinal column. It is vital that the pelvis is aligned and stable, in order to provide the spine with a steady, balanced platform. The muscles of the pelvic girdle are: abdominals, glutes (buttocks), hamstrings (at the back of the thighs), inner thighs and pelvic floor. It is important to tone and strengthen these muscles so that the pelvis remains stable.

Exercises for specific parts of the spine

Neck and upper body: 4–7, 10, 13, 15, 16, 18, 19.

Lower back: 2, 3, 9, 11, 13, 14, 21, 22.

Releasing tension in whole spine: 1–3, 13, 14, 20–24.

LIST
of
EXERCISES

The basic top ten

Stretches

De-rotation

Lengthening

Letting go of the bossy muscle

Teaching the weak side to talk

Pelvic stability

1. REACH FOR THE SKY

Purpose

- Lengthen the spine.

- Stretch and release tight upper back muscles.

Instructions

Repetitions: 3

1. Stand with your feet hip-width apart, arms relaxed by your sides. Float the head upwards and lengthen the spine (as if being stretched like a rubber band).

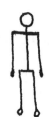

2. Inhale and lift your arms out to the side and then overhead.

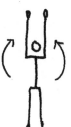

3. Reach your fingertips towards the ceiling, stretching upwards. Then relax, dropping the shoulders away from the ears. Repeat this upward stretch 3 times.

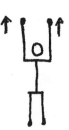

4. Exhale and lower your arms back down to your sides.

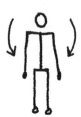

Watch points

- Check your alignment in a mirror if possible. Ensure that your head is not tilted to one side. Check that there is a straight line linking your nose, breast bone, navel, pubic bone and the space between your feet.

- Make sure your weight is equally distributed on both feet.

- Think of floating your rib cage and upper body away from your hips when you make the upward stretch. Try to maximize the distance between your hips and lowest rib, making sure the distance is the same on both sides.

2. SPINE FLEX

Purpose

- Flexible and supple spine.

Instructions

Repetitions: 3

1. Kneel on all fours, with your hands under your shoulders, and knees hip-width apart (like the legs of a coffee table). Keep your neck relaxed and straight.

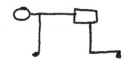

2. Focus now on your tailbone. Raise the tailbone a few centimetres upwards towards the ceiling, then downwards towards the floor. The rest of your spine will move naturally. Don't try to control it, just focus on the vertical line your tailbone is making up and down. Repeat this flowing up-and-down movement 4 times.

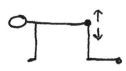

3. Now focus on your upper back at bra strap or breast bone level. Raise this point of the spine upwards a few centimetres, then lower it down towards the floor. (Keep your arms straight and the rest of your spine relaxed.) Repeat this up-and-down movement in flowing motion 4 times.

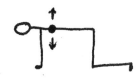

4. Walk your hands forward. Draw your bottom backwards towards the wall behind you (keeping the gentle natural curve in your lower back). Feel the lengthening and stretching of your spine.

Watch points

- Don't brace or grip. Just concentrate on raising and lowering that part of the spine. Let the rest of the spine move naturally, like a string of pearls.

- If your wrists or knees feel strained, place a pillow or folded towel under them.

Modifications

Once you have mastered moving the tailbone and breast bone points, try shifting the focal point to different parts of the spine (e.g. navel or centre back).

Caution

If you have had a spinal fusion operation, or disc problems, check with your doctor before doing this exercise.

3A. FULL BODY STRETCH

Purpose

- Improve spinal flexibility.

- Lengthen the spine.

- A good stretch for the whole body.

Instructions

Repetitions: 3

1. Lie on your back, with straight legs and arms stretched out behind the head.

2. Stretch and lengthen the entire body, reaching the fingertips towards the wall behind the head, and the toes in the opposite direction. Try to maximize the distance between your toes and fingertips.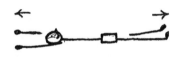

3. Bend one knee and then bring it up to your chest. Hug this knee to your chest with both hands. Hold for a count of 3.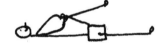

4. Lower the knee and slide the foot and arms back along the floor to starting position. Stretch out the fingertips and toes in opposite directions.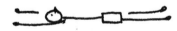

5. Repeat with the other leg (i.e. bend the knee, hug knee to chest for 3 counts, then return to starting position, stretching out arms and legs).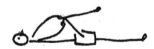

6. Now bring both knees up to the chest (one after the other). Gently hug your knees to your chest, for a count of 3.

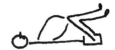

7. Stretch out again to starting position (sliding one foot at a time back along the ground). Feel the full body stretch as you reach fingers and toes in opposite directions. Then relax.

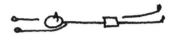

Watch points

- Make sure to slide the foot along the ground when bending your knee, rather than lifting it off the ground straight away. This protects the lumbar spine.

- Do not bend and lift both knees to the chest at the same time. Always move one leg at a time, to protect the lower back.

- If you have a knee problem, clasp the leg under the thigh, rather than on the knee, so that the knee joint is not compressed.

Modifications

When you have mastered this exercise, add 'Foot and hand circles' when stretching out the arms and legs in starting position. 'Foot and hand circles' (exercise 3b) are described on the next page.

3B. FOOT AND HAND CIRCLES

Purpose

- Encourage circulation and flexibility.
- Release tension in wrist and ankle joints.
- Stretch and lengthen the spine.

Instructions

Repetitions: 3

1. Lie on your back with your legs straight, and your arms stretched out behind the head.

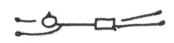

2. Keeping the legs and arms still, rotate the feet and hands, circling from the ankle and wrist joints. Make five circles in one direction.

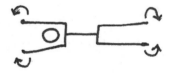

3. Now rotate the hands and feet in the other direction, for five circles.

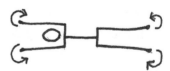

4. Stretch out the body, reaching the fingers and toes in opposite directions. Then relax.

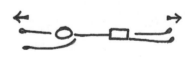

Watch points

- Don't just twiddle the fingers and toes around. Be sure to work from the ankle and wrist joints.

- Try to circle slowly, making the circles as large as you can.

Modifications

Foot and hand circles can be done as a separate exercise, or can be combined with the full body stretch (exercise 3a). Simply add the circles when stretching in start position.

4. WINDMILL

Purpose

- Mobilize the shoulders and upper back.

- Improve shoulder blade stabilization.

- Release tension in the neck, shoulders and upper body.

- Stretch chest muscles to counteract round shoulders.

- Strengthen and tone the back, chest and arm muscles.

Instructions

Repetitions: 6 (3 times each side)

1. Lie on your back, knees bent. Feet are hip-width apart. Arms are straight, pointing up to the ceiling. Palms face towards your knees.

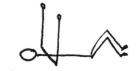

2. Lower your right arm to the floor by your hip. At the same time, take your left arm back behind your head. (The left palm faces the ceiling, the right palm faces the floor.)

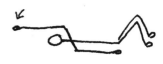

3. Bring both arms back to the start position, pointing towards the ceiling.

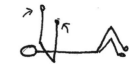

4. Repeat the movement with the opposite arms (i.e. lower the left arm to your hip, and your right arm back behind the head). Return to start position.

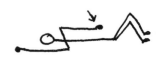

5. Once again, lower your right arm down by your hip and your left arm behind your head.

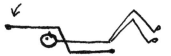

6. Slowly move the arms in an arch close to the floor. Like the arms of a windmill, your arms change places. So now you end up with the left arm by your hip, and the right arm behind your head.

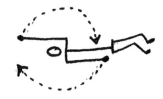

7. Lift both arms up to return to start position.

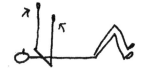

Watch points

- Don't bend your arms, or lift your shoulders towards your ears.

- Don't force your arm all the way back to the floor. Only take your arm back as far as is comfortable, while ensuring that the shoulder blades stay down into your back, and your elbow doesn't bend.

- Go for quality of movement rather than trying to force your arms to touch the floor. Work only within your range.

Modifications

- Place a rolled-up hand towel under your upper back level with your breast bone. This opens the chest.

- If your shoulders and upper spine are very stiff, try reducing the range of movement. Just take your arms half-way in each direction, until you become more flexible.

Caution

If you have a shoulder injury, check with your doctor before doing this exercise.

5. FIGURE OF EIGHT

Purpose

- Release neck tension.

Instructions

Repetitions: 5 each direction

1. Lie on your back with knees bent and arms by your sides. (If necessary, place a folded towel under your head for comfort.)

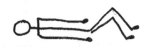

2. Imagine there is a blackboard just above your head, and a piece of chalk on the tip of your nose. You are going to write the figure '8' on the blackboard with your nose.

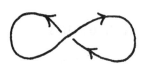

3. Very slowly draw the first loop to one side.

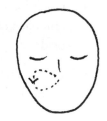

4. Continue the movement by drawing the second loop on the other side with your nose. Finish the figure '8' by bringing your nose back to the centre.

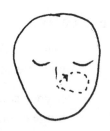

5. Now begin another figure '8' making the movements slow, smooth and continuous.

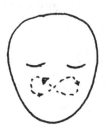

Watch points

- Closing your eyes helps concentration in this exercise.

- Try to make the movement as smooth and flowing as possible. It may feel very jagged at first, but will become smoother as you benefit from the exercise.

- Keep the movement slow. Don't rush.

- Don't strain to make the figure of '8' too large. Keep the movement within your comfort range and quite small.

Modifications

If the figure '8' movement feels complicated, modify the exercise by making a simple circle shape instead.

Caution

Check this exercise with your doctor if you have had a neck injury.

6. ARM PRESSES

Purpose

- Release upper back tension.

- Loosen bunched-up shoulder muscles.

- Strengthen upper back muscles.

- Open up the chest and front.

Instructions

Repetitions: 10

1. Sit on a chair without arms. Feet are flat on the floor, with hips and knees at right angles. Arms are by your sides, with palms facing the wall behind. Check your alignment, lengthen the spine and float the head up.

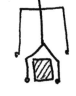

2. Gently push your left palm back (keeping the arm straight). Return your arm to your side.

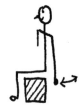

3. Push your right palm back. Then return it to your side.

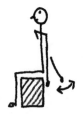

4. Now push both palms back at the same time. (Keep your spine lengthened and your head floating upwards.) Feel the squeeze between your shoulder blades. Return both palms to your side.

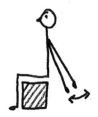

Watch points

- Don't let your head go forward as you take your arms backwards. Think of the head lengthening upwards, towards the ceiling.

- Try to keep your shoulders down.

- Don't tense the neck and shoulders. Keep the back of the neck long.

Modifications

Try this exercise sitting at a computer, or while standing.

7. SHRUGS WITH ARM PRESSES

Purpose

- Mobilize the shoulders.

- Open the chest.

- Strengthen the upper back muscles.

- Release tension in the neck and upper back.

Instructions

Repetitions: 10

1. Sit on a chair with no arms. Hips and knees are at 90 degrees. Arms are straight and loose at your sides, with palms facing in.

2. Shrug both shoulders up towards your ears. Let your arms remain dangling. Then, relax your shoulders back down again.

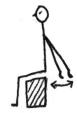

3. Face your palms backwards. Gently push both palms back (keeping the arms straight and the spine and head lengthened). Then return both arms to starting position at your sides.

Watch points

- Don't jerk or jolt the shoulder movements. Make the action soft and gentle. Think of a feather floating down to the ground.

- Don't let the head push forward as you take the palms backwards.

Modifications

Shoulder shrugs can be done alone as a separate exercise. This is good for releasing upper body tension and shoulder mobility.

8. PALMS ON THIGHS PRESS

Purpose

- Lengthen the spine.

- Strengthen the supporting back muscles.

Instructions

Repetitions: Hold for 5 counts. Repeat 3 times

1. Sit on a chair without arms. Feet are flat on the floor, with hips and knees at 90 degrees. Place your palms on your thighs (fingers pointing towards your knees).

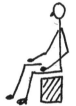

2. Breathe in, then as you breathe out, lengthen the spine upwards as you gently draw your tummy in.

3. Gently press the palms of your hands down on your thighs. (Make sure there is equal pressure on each palm.) Feel the spine lengthen upwards. Hold for 5 counts.

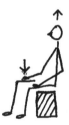

Watch points

- Keep your shoulders down and relaxed.

- Try to keep the length in the spine, at the end of each press.

- Make sure there is equal pressure on each palm.

9. PELVIC ROCKS

Purpose

- Increase spinal flexibility.

- Can relieve lower back stiffness and discomfort.

Instructions

Repetitions: 10

1. Lie on your back, with knees bent at 90 degrees, feet hip-width apart.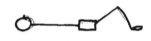

2. Gently rock your pelvis forwards, peeling the tailbone just a few centimetres off the mat, one vertebra at a time. (Imagine the spine as a carpet being rolled up from one end.) Feel your lower back make contact with the floor, as the end of the spine curls upwards.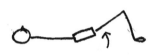

3. Lower the end of the spine back down, one vertebra at a time. Now gently rock the pelvis in the other direction, so that the tailbone presses lightly into the mat, and there is a slight arch in the lower back.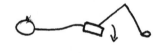

4. Repeat this movement, gently rocking the pelvis forwards and backwards, in a flowing continuous movement.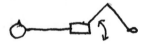

Watch points

- Do not over-arch the spine, or lift the tailbone too high off the mat. Keep the movement small. Arch the back allowing just enough room to slide your fingers between your lower back and the floor.

- Don't tense the neck and shoulders. Try to keep the whole spine relaxed.

10. UPPER BODY RELEASE

Purpose

- Open up chest and counteract hunched shoulders.

- Strengthen muscles in shoulders and between the shoulder blades.

- Excellent for upper body posture.

Instructions

Repetitions: 10

1. Sit on a chair with your elbows bent at right angles, palms facing upwards. Elbows are gently tucked in at the waist.

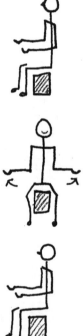

2. Keeping your elbows tucked in at the waist, shift your palms out to the side. Feel your chest open, and your shoulder blades squeeze together.

3. Bring your palms back in front of you, to starting position.

Watch points

- Keep the shoulders down and relaxed, and at equal level.

- Make sure the neck is long and the head is floating upwards.

Modifications

Once you have mastered the 'Upper body release' exercise, try this advanced version:

UPPER BODY RELEASE – ADVANCED VERSION

Instructions

1. Sit on a chair with your elbows bent at right angles. Elbows are gently tucked in at the waist. Your lower arms are out in front of you, with your palms facing inward.

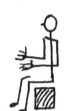

2. Keeping your elbows tucked in at the waist, open your lower arms out to the sides. Feel your chest opening out.

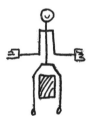

3. When your arms have reached the limit, gently rotate your palms upwards. Now try to shift your hands just a little bit further backwards. (This opens the chest a little more.)

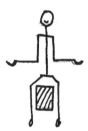

4. Bring your hands back in front of you, and return to starting position.

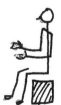

11. HAMSTRING STRETCH

Purpose

- Stretch the hamstring muscles at the back of the thigh.

- Important for alignment and mobility of the lumbar spine.

Instructions

Repetitions: Hold for 1 minute each leg

1. Lie on the floor with both legs bent.

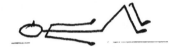

2. Bend the right knee to your chest. Place a scarf or strap over the sole of the foot (holding the scarf in both hands).

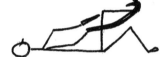

3. Slowly straighten the leg into the air, stretching through your right heel and ball of your foot.

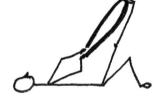

4. Hold the stretch for 1 minute, then repeat with the other leg.

5. To increase the stretch, straighten the other leg, so that it lies flat on the floor.

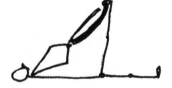

Watch points

- Don't force your leg. Stretch gently within your limits.

- Don't allow your pelvis to twist. Keep the hip bones level on both sides.

- Keep your tailbone down on the mat.

- Make sure the upper body, neck and shoulders are relaxed.

Modifications

Instead of using a scarf, there are other ways of stretching the hamstring:

ALTERNATIVE HAMSTRING STRETCH 1

Instructions

1. Find a doorway where you can stretch one leg up the wall, and lie the other out straight on the floor.

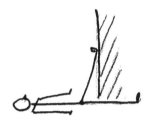

2. Adjust this stretch by: shifting your bottom closer to, or further away from, the door frame; flexing the foot more; bending or straightening the supporting leg.

ALTERNATIVE HAMSTRING STRETCH 2

Instructions

1. Lie on your back, both knees bent. Raise your left knee to your chest and clasp both hands behind it.

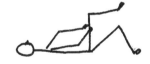

2. Straighten the left leg up into the air. If you can, gently pull it a little towards your chest.

3. Flex and point the foot 5 times. Lower the leg. Repeat with the other leg.

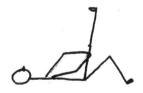

12. HIP FLEXOR STRETCH

Purpose

- Stretch out the hip flexor, quad and psoas muscles at the front of the hip and the thigh.

- Good for lumbar spine stiffness and alignment.

Instructions

Repetitions: Hold for 30–60 seconds each side

1. Kneel in front of a chair. Place your left foot in front of you so that your knee is at 90 degrees over your ankle. Lengthen through your torso, floating the head to the ceiling. (If necessary, hold onto the chair for balance.)

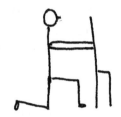

2. Gently shift your torso forward, keeping it vertical. Feel the stretch in the front of the thigh and hip.

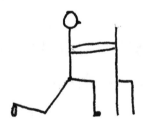

3. To increase the stretch, raise both arms straight above the head. Reach gently upwards.

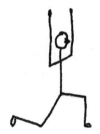

Watch points

- Don't let one hip move further forward than the other. Keep both hips aligned, parallel to the facing wall.

- Keep your shoulders square, and parallel to the wall in front.

- Lengthen the spine and head upwards, with your torso vertical.

- Put a pillow under the knee for protection and comfort, if needed.

- Use the chair for balance, if needed.

Caution

Do not do this exercise if you have knee problems.

13. CAT STRETCH

Purpose

- Stretch and mobilize the spine.

Instructions

Repetitions: 3 times, then rest position

1. Kneel on all fours. Your hands are under your shoulders. Knees are hip-width apart. Your neck is relaxed and straight.

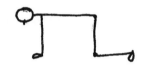

2. Curve your spine upwards, so that the mid back lifts towards the ceiling, like a cat stretching. The head and tailbone drop downwards.

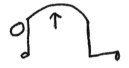

3. Now gently lower the mid back downwards into a slight arch. Your head and tailbone are lifted upwards. Repeat both stretches 3 times.

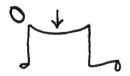

4. Move to the rest position. Shift your tailbone back so that your bottom is on or near your heels. Your arms are stretched out in front. Rest your head on the floor. Walk your fingers forward for a stronger stretch. Hold this position for 1 minute.

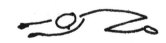

Watch points

- Don't arch your back downwards too far. Make only a gentle small arch.

- If you have wrist or knee discomfort, place a pillow or folded towel under your wrists and knees. If there is still discomfort, miss this exercise.

Modifications

Once you have mastered the basic cat stretch, try adding the following variations to the exercise:

CAT STRETCH WITH ARM EXTENSION

Purpose

- Stabilize and strengthen the torso.

- Stretch and mobilize the spine.

Instructions

1. Kneel on all fours. Your hands are under your shoulders. Knees are hip-width apart. Take a breath in.

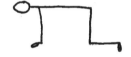

2. As you breathe out, engage your abdominals, and extend your right arm out in front of you. Try to hold your arm at shoulder level without losing your balance, and keeping your torso stable.

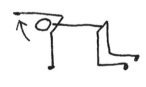

3. Return to start position. Repeat with other arm.

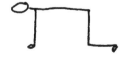

4. Now do the basic cat stretch as described on p.70. Curve the spine upwards, so that the mid back lifts towards the ceiling.

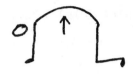

5. Now lower the mid back downwards.

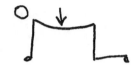

6. Move to the rest position. Shift your tailbone back so that your bottom is on or near your heels. Your arms are stretched out in front.

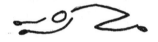

CAT STRETCH WITH TAILBONE SHIFT SIDEWAYS

Purpose

- Encourage flexibility in lumbar spine.

- Stretch and mobilize the spine.

Instructions

1. Kneel on all fours, with hands under your shoulders, and knees hip-width apart.

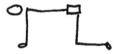

2. Focus on your tailbone. Shift your tailbone a few centimetres across to the right, then back to centre.

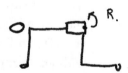

3. Now shift your tailbone to the left a few centimetres, then return to centre. Think of drawing a short horizontal line from left to right with the tailbone. Repeat this side-to-side movement in flowing motion 3 times.

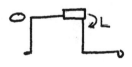

4. Return to the starting position, and do the basic cat stretch exercise.

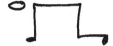

Caution

If you have a lumbar curve and experience discomfort doing this movement, avoid this exercise.

14. PUPPY POSE

Purpose

- Stretch and lengthen the spine.

- Release tension in the upper and lower back.

Instructions

Repetitions: Hold for 30 seconds. Repeat 3 times

1. Kneel on all fours, hands forward of the shoulders. Toes are curled under. The lower back is gently arched.

2. Move your bottom back over the heels, keeping the gentle lumbar arch and your tailbone pointing upwards.

3. Press down through the hands, and gently draw your bottom further backwards. Feel the stretch of the spine.

Modifications

Combine this exercise with exercise 25 'Breathing into sunken side'. As you stretch out and lengthen the spine, breathe into the sunken side (i.e. the compressed ribs and waist). This creates space and awareness in the weak area.

15. CHEST OPENING

Purpose

- Open up the chest and shoulders.

- Counteract hunching of the upper body.

Instructions

Repetitions: 3

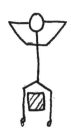

1. Sit on a chair. Fingers are interlinked behind the head.

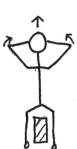

2. Lengthen your spine and head upwards. Gently stretch your elbows backwards, towards the wall behind you. Hold for 10 seconds.

Watch points

- Don't force the elbows backwards. Stretch only to 80 per cent of your capacity.

- Don't let the head move forward (as the elbows go back).

- Keep the head and neck lengthened and relaxed.

- Keep your shoulders down.

Caution

If you have shoulder problems, check with your doctor before doing this exercise.

16. COSSACK ARMS

Purpose

- Rotation of the spine, with stability and strength.

Instructions

Repetitions: 10 each side

1. Sit up straight, with your elbows out at the sides, and your palms facing downwards. Touch your fingertips together in front of your breast bone. Relax your shoulders and neck completely. Lengthen your spine and head upwards.

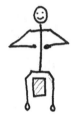

2. Gently turn your upper body round to the right. (Keep your nose and fingertips in line with your breast bone.) Make sure your hips and knees are still, and equally weighted. Don't try to turn too far.

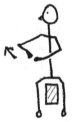

3. Return to the centre, starting position. Repeat on the other side.

Watch points

- Don't move your hips or knees. Try to keep them as still as possible. Put a pillow between the knees, if needed.

- Don't lean or sink to one side. Try to keep equal weight on both buttocks, and also on both feet.

- Make sure your shoulders are down and level.

- Keep lengthening and floating the head towards the ceiling throughout the exercise.

- Don't turn the head too far. It should move naturally and stay in line with your fingertips.

Caution

Consult your doctor before doing this exercise if you have a disc-related injury or operation.

17. ONE-ARM COSSACK

Purpose

- Help mobilize the middle of your back.

- Rotation of the spine.

Instructions

Repetitions: 10 each side

1. Sit upright on a chair with your fingertips touching at breast bone level. Palms face downwards.

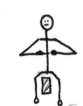

2. Gently rotate your upper body to the right.

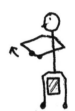

3. Stretch your right arm out straight to your side. Gently push it backwards, rotating it even more.

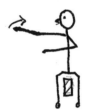

4. Bend your right arm in, so that your finger-tips touch again. Return to centre.

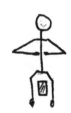

5. Repeat on the other side.

Watch points

- Don't lean or sink to one side. Keep your hips and feet equally weighted.

- Try to keep your lower body still. Don't move your hips and knees. If necessary, place a cushion between the knees.

- Make sure your shoulders are down and level.

- Keep lengthening your spine, neck and head upwards.

Modifications

If you have difficulty holding your arms up in 'Cossack' position, replace this exercise with number 18 'Straight arm rotation'.

18. STRAIGHT ARM ROTATION

Purpose

- Gentle rotation of the spine.

Instructions

Repetitions: 10 each side

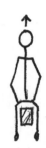

1. Sit on a chair, with your hands resting on your thighs. Lengthen the spine and head upwards.

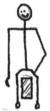

2. Take one arm down by your side, palm facing inwards.

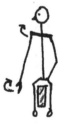

3. Keeping your arms straight, gently rotate your arm and hand towards the wall behind you. Imagine your thumb tracing a semi-circle or an arch shape (about 30 cm wide). As you rotate, your thumb points first to the front, then to the side wall and then to the wall behind. Let your upper body turn to the side as your hand moves.

4. Hold the rotated position for 3 counts. Return to start position. Repeat on other side.

Watch points

- Keep your shoulder blades down and your shoulders level.

- Let your head and upper body turn naturally as you rotate the arm backwards.

- Don't sink or lean to one side. Try to keep weight equal on both sides.

- Keep your lower body still, with no movement of hips or knees.

- Don't force your arm backwards. Work within a comfortable range of movement.

19A. LENGTH AWARENESS – GROWING TALLER

Purpose

- Create an awareness of spinal lengthening.

- Improve posture.

Instructions

Repetitions: 3

1. Stand or sit in front of a mirror. Place the palm of your hand about 1 cm above your head.

2. Float your head upwards, trying to touch your hand. Feel the spine lengthening, and keep that length (rather than relaxing back down).

3. Repeat the exercise (moving your hand up 1 cm above your head's new position and growing your head upwards to touch your hand again).

4. Now do the same head lengthening exercise, this time with both hands by your sides. Concentrate simply on lengthening the head and spine upwards, growing taller each time.

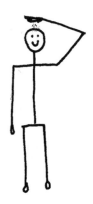

Watch points

- Don't tilt your head backwards, by raising the chin and arching the back of your neck. Think of floating the whole head upwards like a balloon.

- This exercise is great for posture awareness. It can be done anywhere, sitting or standing, especially when you catch yourself slumping.

19B. LENGTH AWARENESS – SHOULDERS DOWN

Purpose

- Length awareness.
- Improve posture.

Instructions

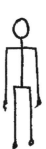

Repetitions: 3

1. Sit or stand with your arms by your sides, palms facing in.

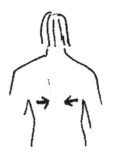

2. Squeeze your shoulder blades together, trying to get them to touch.

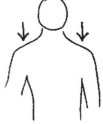

3. Bring your shoulders down and really relax them. (Imagine your shoulders blades sinking to the floor.)

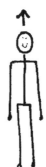

4. Relax the neck. Float the head up. Feel your whole spine being stretched like a rubber band.

20. PUPPY POSE WITH HAND SLIDE

Purpose

- Lengthen the spine.

- Stretch out tight back muscles.

Instructions

Repetitions: 3

1. Kneel on the floor with your arms straight out in front. Your palms are flat on the floor (fingers pointing forwards).

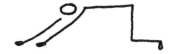

2. Make a gentle arch in your lower back, by pointing your tailbone slightly upwards.

3. Move your bottom backwards over your heels.

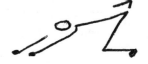

4. Slide your hands forward along the floor. Then gently shift your bottom backwards again, feeling the stretch in your spine. (Allow your hands to shift a little along the floor as you move your bottom backwards.)

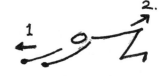

5. Hold the stretch for the count of 3.

6. Repeat steps 3 to 5, alternately moving your bottom backwards and then shifting your palms forwards.

Watch points

- This is the same basic exercise as number 14, 'Puppy pose', only with hands shifting forwards along the ground, for extra lengthening.

- Make sure that there is equal pressure on both hands. (There may be a tendency to favour the hand of the dominant strong side.)

Modifications

- Combine this exercise with number 25, 'Breathing into sunken side'. As you stretch out the spine, breathe into the sunken side (i.e. the compressed ribs and waist). This creates space and awareness in the weak side.

- Move the hands forward on a roller, instead of sliding your palms along the floor, as described below. Any long cylindrical object with a 10–20 cm diameter will work as a roller (e.g. a roll of wallpaper or a piece of PVC pipe).

PUPPY POSE WITH ROLLER

Instructions

1. Kneel on the floor, with your arms straight out in front, your hands on the roller.

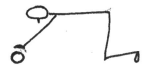

2. Make a gentle arch in your lower back, by pointing your tailbone slightly upwards.

3. Move your bottom backwards over your heels. At the same time, roll your hands forward on the roller. Feel your spine lengthening like a rubber band, as your bottom moves backwards and your hands reach forwards.

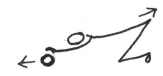

4. Hold the stretch for the count of 3. (For more stretch, roll the hands a little further forward again.) Gently return to start position.

21. BACKWARDS PULL

Purpose

- Stretch and lengthen the spine.

Instructions

Repetitions: Hold for 5 counts. Repeat 3 times

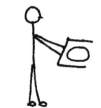

1. Stand in front of a kitchen sink or a fixed vertical pole. Feet are hip-width apart. Hold the pole or sink with both hands.

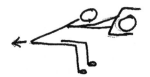

2. Bend your knees to 90 degrees and gently pull back with your hips. Let the weight of your body fall backwards to your bottom. Make sure to hold on firmly with your hands. Hold for 5 counts.

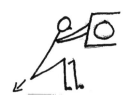

3. A variation of this stretch: Walk the feet forward a few inches. Drop your bottom to a squat and gently pull your bottom backwards, stretching the lower back. Hold for 5 counts.

22. PHYSIO BALL STRETCH

Purpose

- Stretch and lengthen the spine.

Instructions

Repetitions: Hold for 5 counts. Repeat 3 times

1. Get a chair and ask someone to sit firmly on the seat to stabilize it.

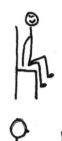

2. Sit on the centre of the physio ball, facing the chair. Hold firmly onto each side of the chair with your hands. Your hands should be roughly in line with your armpits.

3. Roll backwards, letting your bottom curve over the ball, and your feet lift off the ground. Relax your shoulders and neck. Feel the stretch along the length of your spine, as your weight falls down towards your bottom. Hold for 5 counts.

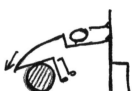

4. Slowly return to start position.

Watch points

Choose a physio ball the right size. When you sit, your bottom should be at the same level or slightly higher than your knees.

23. MASSAGE BALL ON WALL

Purpose

- Relax and release tightness in the bossy muscle area.

Instructions

Repetitions: Massage each point for about 10 counts

1. Take a tennis ball or massage ball. (This is a plastic ball with small spikes, sometimes called 'Noppen ball' or 'spiky ball'.)

2. Stand with your back close to a wall, knees slightly bent.

3. Place the ball on the tight muscle area. Lean back towards the wall, so that the ball is sandwiched between your back and the wall. (Your back does not touch the wall.)

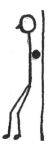

4. Relax the weight of your body onto the ball. Massage the tight part of your back against the ball (by moving slightly from side to side). Focus on that point for about 10 counts.

5. Shift the ball to massage other parts of your back that are tight and tense.

Watch points

- Move your back against the ball by bending your knees and shifting gently from side to side.

- Keep the head and spine lengthened upwards throughout.

- Don't put the ball on the bones of the spine. Work on the muscles on either side of the vertebrae.

- This exercise can be done sitting on a chair to release tight muscles, if you have to sit for a long time.

24. RELAXATION POSE

Purpose

* Relax the whole spine and back muscles.

Instructions

Do this at the end of an exercise session
Repetitions: Stay in the pose for 2–3 minutes

1. Lie on a firm comfortable surface or mat. Place a couple of pillows under your knees so that your legs are bent and relaxed. Arms are relaxed out to the sides with palms facing up. (You can place a folded hand towel under the bossy muscle to raise it slightly, if you wish.)

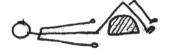

2. Close your eyes. Concentrate on your breathing. Allow your back to lengthen and widen. Let your back relax into the mat with each out breath.

25. BREATHING INTO SUNKEN SIDE

Purpose

- Encourage awareness of the weak area, through stimulus and breath.

- Increase lung capacity in the weak side.

- Open and lengthen the sunken side of the torso.

Instructions

Repetitions: 10 each day

1. Place the palm of your hand on the sunken part of your back. If you can't reach this point with your hand, ask a friend to put their hand on this area.

2. Imagine an empty glass or an empty balloon in that area of your body.

3. Breathe into this area. Imagine filling up the balloon or glass with your breath. Make sure to breathe slowly and deeply. Inhale through your nose and exhale through your mouth.

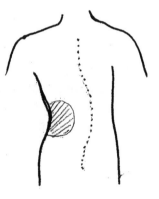

4. Feel the handprint area on your back open and expand with your breath.

Watch points

- This exercise can be done sitting or standing.

- Once you are confident with the location of the handprint area, you can do the exercise without placing the hand on your back.

Modifications

- Combine this exercise with number 14, 'Puppy pose', for extra length and opening.

- The same exercise can be done lying down:

BREATHING INTO SUNKEN SIDE – LYING DOWN

Purpose

- Helps to concentrate breathing on the weak side of your lungs.

- Opens and lengthens the sunken side of the torso.

Instructions

Repetitions: 10

1. Position a stool next to you. Then, lie with your 'flat waist', 'bossy muscle' side on the floor. Extend your lower arm along the floor. Place one pillow under your ribs, and another between your head and lower arm.

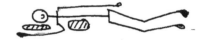

2. Stretch your upper arm over your head, so that your hand touches the seat of the stool.

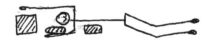

3. Breathe into your weak sunken side. Imagine filling up a balloon on that side with your breath.

4. Breathe out, and try to keep a little space and openness in the sunken area. Take 3 deep breaths, in and out. Release your arm back down.

26. ONE-ARM ARCH

Purpose

- Strengthen the muscles on the weak side.

Instructions

Repetitions: 10 on weak side

1. Lie on your back with knees bent, feet hip-width apart. Arms are straight up, with your hands in line with the breast bone. Palms face inwards.

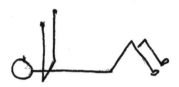

2. Breathe into your sunken side and keep this space and length.

3. Open the arm of your sunken side out to the side. Imagine you are repainting the arc of half a rainbow, beginning at the centre and working your way out to the end of the rainbow, near the floor.

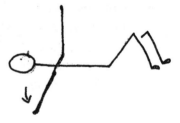

4. Return your arm up to start position, using the lateral muscles under your arm.

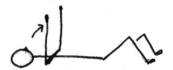

Watch points

- Keep your shoulder blades down and relaxed. Don't let them move up towards your ears when you open your arm out to the side.

- Make sure your arm stays slightly curved, with the elbow bent at the same gentle angle throughout.

- Try to keep your hand in line with the armpit as you make the arch. Don't allow it to creep up towards your chin.

Modifications

Combine this 'one arm arch' exercise with 'two arm arches' where you make arches with both arms simultaneously.

27. ONE-ARM PRESS ON WALL

Purpose

- Strengthen the muscles on the weak side.

Instructions

Repetitions: 10 on weak side

1. Place a stool in a doorway. Position it so that the shoulder of your weak side is slightly in front of, and in line with, the door frame.

2. The arm of your weak side is straight down by your side, with the palm facing backwards. Lengthen the spine upwards. Breathe into the sunken side (and keep this space and length throughout the exercise).

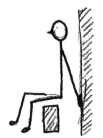

3. Move the palm of your hand backwards, so that it presses gently against the door frame. Hold for 3 counts, then relax.

Watch points

- Don't sink down into the sunken side. Make sure to keep the space and length in this weak area.

- Keep your shoulders down and relaxed. Try not to brace or grip. Make the movement gentle.

- Try to keep lengthening the head and spine throughout.

Modifications

This exercise can also be done standing up.

28. ONE-ARM SLIDES ON WALL

Purpose

- Strengthen muscles on the weak sunken side.

Instructions

Repetitions: 10 on weak side

1. Stand with your weak side towards a wall. Bend your elbow at 90 degrees, and place your forearm on the wall, palm facing forwards. Your elbow, forearm and little finger are touching the wall.

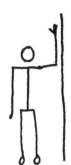

2. To prepare, breathe into the sunken side, and lengthen your spine and head upwards. Keep the space and length in the sunken side.

3. Gently slide your forearm down the wall, using the muscles under your arm.

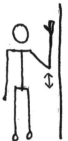

4. Now slide the forearm back up the wall to start position.

Watch points

Make sure your shoulders are down and relaxed. Don't let them brace or shift upwards.

29. LYING ON SIDE WITH PAD

Purpose

- Stretch and lengthen the weak sunken side.

- Encourage breathing in the compressed ribs or waist.

Instructions

Repetitions: Hold for 1 minute

1. Lie on your bossy muscle side (the side with a rib hump or straight waist). Your knees are bent.

2. Place a rolled-up towel or a bolster under your side, at the arch point of the major curve.

3. Reach the upper arm overhead. Hold the wrist of the upper arm with opposite hand.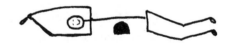

4. Breathe into the sunken area, compressed ribs or waist.

30. GLUTE SQUEEZES

Purpose

- Connect and strengthen the glute (buttock) muscles.

Instructions

Repetitions: 10

1. Lie face down on the floor with a folded towel between your thighs. Place a pillow under your tummy. Rest your forehead on your hands. When you're ready, breathe in.

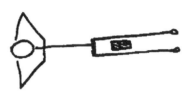

2. As you breathe out, gently draw your tummy in. Squeeze your buttocks towards each other. Hold the squeeze for 4 counts. Then release.

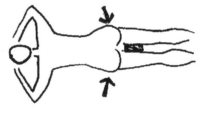

Watch points

- Be sure to squeeze each buttock equally. There can be a tendency with scoliosis for one side to dominate.

- Relax the upper body. Make sure your neck and shoulders do not tense up.

- The lower legs and feet are also relaxed. Only the buttocks and abs are doing the work.

31. ABDOMINAL DRAWING-IN

Purpose

- Gentle abdominal connection without straining the neck or back.

Instructions

Repetitions: 5 each side

1. Lie on your side with your knees bent. Extend your lower arm under your head. Put a pillow between your lower arm and head for support.

2. Place the hand of your upper arm over your stomach. Your hand will cradle the curved shape of your relaxed abdomen. Let your stomach hang down towards the floor. (Don't worry about the bulge of your stomach. Everyone has it when they lie on their side and relax their abs. It's gravity!)

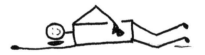

3. Breathe in deeply. Then, as you breathe out, pull your stomach up first and then backwards, away from your hand. Keep it contracted away from your hand for the count of 5. Then relax.

4. Once you've mastered this, try holding the abdominal contraction for longer, as you breathe from the chest.

Watch points

- Keep the rest of your body still. Only the abdominals move in this exercise. Your spine and torso remain relaxed and still. Be careful not to flatten the lower back as you contract your abs.

- Place a folded towel under your waist when lying on your dominant side with a straight waist. A towel is not necessary when you lie on the sunken curved waist side.

32. HAMSTRING CURLS

Purpose

* Connect and strengthen the hamstring muscles (at the back of the thighs).

Instructions

Repetitions: 10 each side

1. Lie face down on the floor with a pillow under your tummy. Rest your forehead on your hands. Stretch each leg a little and make sure your legs are straight and parallel. Breathe in.

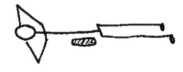

2. As you breathe out, very slowly bend your right leg, until your knee is at a right angle, i.e. raise your heel towards your buttocks. Your foot is relaxed, with the sole of the foot towards the ceiling. You may feel the muscles at the back of the thigh working.

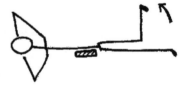

3. Lower the foot back to the ground. Repeat 10 times with each leg.

Watch points

* It's important to raise your heel in a straight line towards your buttocks. Imagine a direct line from your buttock to your heel, and don't waver from it.

* If possible, ask someone to check your alignment, to make sure that your body and legs are straight, and that you're keeping the heel to buttock straight line.

33. INNER THIGH SQUEEZE

Purpose

- Connect and strengthen the inner thigh (adductor) muscles.

Instructions

Repetitions: Hold for 4 counts. Repeat 10 times

1. Lie on your back with your knees bent and feet hip-width apart. Place a pillow between your knees. Relax your upper body into the floor. Breathe in.

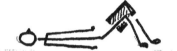

2. As you breathe out, engage your abdominals. Then gently squeeze the cushion with your inner thighs. Don't grip too hard. Hold for the count of 4. Then release.

Watch points

- Your upper body remains totally relaxed. Be sure that it doesn't move, or take any tension.

- Make the exercise a slow gentle squeeze, without any jerking movement.

34. PELVIC FLOOR

Purpose

- Engage and strengthen the pelvic floor (see note below).

Instructions

Repetitions: Hold for 5 counts. Repeat 10 times

1. Sit on a chair with your knees as far apart as is comfortable. Your feet are flat on the floor. Lean forward from the waist. Place your hands on your knees to support your back and keep it straight. Keep your shoulders down and relaxed.

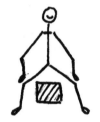

2. Now, imagine that you are pulling your bladder toward your rib cage. Feel the internal lift of this movement. Hold for 5 counts. Then release.

Note

The pelvic floor muscles, which form a hammock or sling shape between your legs, help to hold your pelvis in correct alignment. To identify the pelvic floor muscles, imagine that you are trying to prevent the flow of urine, or that you are walking into an icy cold pool of water.

WHAT EXERCISES TO AVOID

Gentle, inner-range exercise on a regular basis is beneficial for scoliosis. It encourages flexibility, lengthening and muscle tone. On the other hand, there are certain exercises to avoid, especially for those individuals whose scoliosis is more severe. It is wise to steer clear of the following exercise movements, or at least to check with a physical therapist and do them under supervision.

- **Bending and twisting** at the same time.

- **Heavy weight-bearing exercise.** Using weights that are too heavy will cause the body to brace and the spine to compress. It is far better to use lighter weights and do more repetitions.

- **High-impact exercise** that involves jumping, jolting or jarring movements which compress the spine (e.g. jogging on hard surfaces).

- **Excessive outer-range movements.** Keep within a comfortable range of movement. Work at 80 per cent of your full range and keep the movement gentle and flowing. Listen to your body and be aware of what it's telling you. Outer-range movement is fine for athletes and dancers, but with scoliosis it is far better to start with smaller, gentle, inner-range movements, and then gradually work towards outer-range as your body permits.

- **Extreme flexion and extension of the spine.** It's fine to flex and extend the spine through small, gentle inner-range movements. However, do not overdo it. Avoid extreme outer-range curving or arching the back. This places undue pressure and strain on the spine.

- **Repeated lateral or sideways bending** without supervision. Scoliosis involves a lateral curve of the spine. Repeated bending sideways into the curve (i.e. towards the sunken side) will promote the curvature and encourage the asymmetry of the torso. For this reason, side-bending should be done only under the advice of a physical therapist who understands the structure of your particular curvature.

- **Excessive exertion, bracing or gripping.** When we are fatigued or trying too hard in an exercise, the body braces itself and old patterns of muscle connection and unbalanced alignment kick in; in other words the old dominant muscle pattern takes over. So, don't try too hard, don't overdo any exercise, and stop before you become fatigued.

- **Pelvic twisting or rotation** if you have a lumbar curve. In lumbar scoliosis, the pelvis is usually misaligned, with one hip higher and/or further forward than the other. It is important to align and stabilize the pelvis. Thus it is wise to avoid sideways twisting movements or rotation of the pelvis without supervision.

- **Excessive 'navel-to-spine' abdominal contraction.** Quite often in exercise classes you hear the catch-cry 'pull your navel towards your spine and draw your tummy in!' This is fine, as long as you *do not flatten your lower back* in the process. Always aim for a gentle natural curve in your lower back. (This is sometimes called 'neutral spine'.) Excessive and repetitive back flattening through abdominal contraction may, over time, result in spinal strain, compression and hunched posture in the upper body. If you want to strengthen your abdominal muscles, do the 'Abdominal drawing-in' exercise (number 31).

POSSIBLE GOALS AND OUTCOMES

'Can exercise help my scoliosis?' 'What can I expect to achieve?'

These questions are frequently asked and strongly debated. Some claim that exercise is ineffective as it does not 'cure' scoliosis (Schommer 2002), while others provide strong evidence of positive results of a systematic, individually tailored exercise programme for scoliosis (Lehnert-Schroth 2007; Weiss 2006). The following case study describes what I have found in my own particular case of scoliosis.

Case study

When I was 37, I began a gentle exercise programme (in the form of walking, swimming, rehabilitation Pilates and yoga) because I was aware of my scoliosis becoming more hunched, severe and painful. By this time, my spine was rigid and my torso was increasingly twisted. I realized that I needed to do something and to explore options, instead of passively sitting by and lamenting the 'degeneration' of my spine. Over the next ten years, I included the gentle exercise programme in my everyday lifestyle. These are the outcomes:

- Increased flexibility of the spine (in both the thoracic and lumbar areas).

- Reduced protrusion of the rib cage at the front, and reduced rib hump on the back.

- Shoulder blade winging is markedly less.

- Shoulder alignment is now equal (i.e. one shoulder is no longer higher than the other).

- Muscle tone is much improved. The dominant muscle block is still evident, but less rigid and strained. The weaker sunken side now has some muscle development. However, the asymmetrical muscle pattern is still quite evident.

- Posture and alignment is greatly improved. Kyphosis (hunching and stooping forward) of the upper body, and lordosis (overarching backwards) of the lumbar spine, have reduced markedly.

- Back pain has dramatically reduced in both the upper and lower back. Discomfort and pain does return when I miss a few days of flexibility exercises.

- There has been no change in the degree or size of the lateral curvature. The lateral curve remains at 38 degrees to the left between T6 and T10, and at 60 degrees to the right from T10 to L5. In short, the size of the curve has not decreased, nor has it progressed.

Summarizing, while the degree of the lateral curvature has remained the same, there have been marked positive changes in posture and alignment, spinal flexibility, rib cage protrusion, muscle tone and strength, and pain and discomfort levels.

MORE ABOUT PILATES

This section is for those readers who would like to learn more about the Pilates method. We look in more detail at Pilates and its basic principles, how it was created by Joseph Pilates, and how Pilates for scoliosis differs from a general Pilates programme.

About the Pilates method

Pilates is a gentle form of exercise, helping your mind and body to work in harmony to produce a healthy, toned, mobile body and a calm, relaxed mind. Using posture and breathing as key elements, Pilates is a non-aerobic exercise method for lengthening and strengthening the muscles, and encouraging flexibility. Essentially, Pilates is not a rigid set regime. Rather it is constantly adjusted and moulded to suit the particular needs of the individual. Key concepts and principles of the Pilates method are:

- **Breathing.** Focus is on deep relaxed rhythmic breathing in cadence with the flow of movement. Awareness of the breath is vital. Proper breathing means that the blood can be charged with oxygen and can do its work efficiently, awakening the body's cells. Generally in Pilates, movement with effort is made on the out breath.

- **Focus and concentration.** It is important to focus the mind clearly on the movement and position of the body. Complete attention is given to the movement, keeping the mind on the present moment and letting go of other thoughts as they appear. Listening to your breath and feeling the movement is vital. This enables mind–body awareness and is also profoundly relaxing!

- **Centring.** One of the basic aims of Pilates is to strengthen the deep core muscles. The idea is to protect the spine and create a strong base for you to carry out ordinary movements. Centring is vital for your every movement, whether you are out walking or sitting at a desk. Your 'centre' is the continuous band of muscles stretching around your body between the bottom of your rib cage and across your hip bones. This centre is sometimes referred to as 'core stability'. If these muscles are weak, the back is much more vulnerable to injury, strain and pelvic instability.

- **Flowing movement.** Pilates exercises aim for continuous fluid movement. One position flows as gently and naturally as possible into the next. Try not to strain, or to move too stiffly or jerkily.

- **Control and isolation of muscles.** A distinguishing feature of Pilates is the isolation of muscle groups – you learn to move and engage individual muscle groups, while keeping the rest of the body aligned and relaxed.

- **Individualization.** Each body is different and each of us has different needs and abilities. Learning how to do Pilates helps us to build up an awareness of our own individual body. A good Pilates programme will enhance this body awareness by constantly adjusting to suit individual progress and needs.

- **Relaxation and letting go.** It is vital to let go of any tendency to strain, brace the body, or try too hard while doing Pilates exercises. Focus is on relaxed, natural and effortless movement.

- **Precision.** Carrying out the movements as mindfully and exactly as you can will have more impact and more lasting value. It creates a feeling of fine-tuning the body, and this state is then echoed in your life as grace and ease of movement.

About Joseph Pilates

The Pilates exercise regime was devised by Joseph Pilates (1880–1967). Born near Dusseldorf in Germany, he was a frail and sickly child suffering from asthma, rickets and rheumatic fever. Determined to overcome his fragility, he experimented with many different approaches including yoga, gymnastics, skiing, self-defence, dance and weight-training. Selecting the effective aspects of these diverse methods, Pilates created his unique and evolving system of health and physical fitness.

In 1912, Pilates shifted to England, working as a professional boxer and self-defence instructor to detectives in Scotland Yard. During World War One, Pilates was interned in England where he worked as a nurse to the other inmates. Many needed physical therapy, including war veterans with severe injuries and amputations. Pilates experimented with springs attached to the walls over beds to allow patients to rehabilitate while lying on their backs. In this way patients could work on muscle strength, and it was noticed they improved faster than others.

After the war, Pilates returned to Germany briefly where he continued working on his fitness regime. In 1926 he emigrated to the USA and set up his first studio in New York. The Pilates method gained immediate success among dancers and gymnasts who recognized its value in their training and rehabilitation. At the time of his death, the Pilates method was still relatively unknown, but has since found a far wider audience.

Over the decades since Joseph Pilates set up his studio, his technique has been developed in a variety of ways. Like the disciplines of yoga and Tai Chi, there are now a range of different types of Pilates. For example, some teachers focus on intense fast-paced movement, while in other forms of Pilates, movement is extremely gentle, slow and rhythmic allowing weaker muscles to be located and well worked.

Pilates for scoliosis

The Pilates exercises in this book have been specifically tailored to suit people with scoliosis. These are essentially gentle exercises for flexibility, posture and muscle strength for individuals who have curvature of the spine. The exercises are based on five basic principles:

1. lengthening and flexibility of the spine

2. de-rotation of the spine, ribs and pelvis

3. teaching the bossy dominant muscles to let go

4. teaching the weak side how to talk

5. pelvic stability.

The Pilates for scoliosis exercises in this book differ from a general Pilates programme in that special focus is given to:

- **Gentle inner-range movement.** It is important to avoid excessive outer-range movement such as extreme curving or arching the back. This places undue pressure and strain on the spine.

- **Alignment of the body.** Keep this as symmetrical as possible. Before beginning the exercise, it is important to put the body in the best possible symmetrical balanced posture, and to maintain this alignment throughout the exercise. Be mindful of the tendency to want to fall back into old asymmetrical posture and movement patterns.

- **Lengthening of the spine,** to avoid contraction and slumping into the scoliotic curve.

- **Engaging the pelvic floor, instead of emphasizing 'navel-to-spine'.** Drawing up the pelvic floor encourages the spine to lengthen and remain supple. In contrast, for people with scoliosis, excessive navel-to-spine abdominal contraction may result in spinal strain and compression, with a tendency to lumbar flat back and hunching forward in the upper body.

- **Isolation of muscle groups.** For people with scoliosis, the Pilates concept of muscle isolation is important. You learn to move and engage separate muscle groups, while keeping the rest of the body aligned and relaxed. In effect, this enables 'rewiring' of the body by teasing out asymmetrical patterns of muscle use. It encourages the building up of weak underdeveloped muscles, and breaks down the tendency for the dominant bossy muscles to do all the work.

With Pilates for scoliosis, the following movements are avoided:

- Bending and twisting at the same time.

- Repeated lateral and sideways bending without supervision.

- Extreme flexion and extension of the spine.

- Pelvic twisting and rotation without supervision if you have a lumbar curve.

- Straining and trying too hard, which only reinforces the torsion of the curve, causing the spine to contract and buckle even more.

It is important to highlight that these exercises are not designed to re-structure the curve. Their purpose is to encourage flexibility and length, and to enable the spine to be as healthy and supple as possible. They are suited for people with all types of scoliosis and can be modified accord-ing to the individual's specific needs. (As mentioned in the introductory pages, it is advisable to check with your doctor before embarking on any exercise programme.)

If you have access to a Pilates studio, a piece of equipment called the 'reformer' is particularly useful for people with scoliosis. The reformer looks like a low flat bed with springs and ropes attached. It enables gentle safe work on muscle strength and alignment, while lying on your back in a relaxed non-strained position.

With the increasing popularity of Pilates, there are a wide range of classes available. These range from mat classes for a large group with quite vigorous outer-range movements, to one-on-one sessions of gentle exercises in a fully equipped studio. For scoliosis, a gentle rehabilitation Pilates programme taught on a one-to-one basis is recommended.

PART 3

Strategies

FOR

Living

WITH

Scoliosis

DIET

A healthy balanced diet is vital for the well-being of people with scoliosis. It is important to keep your body functioning in tip-top condition, fuelling it with good food that enables you to get the maximum benefit and use from your physical structure. If you clog up your body with junk food, it will not function well and physical weaknesses and problems will appear.

Make sure you have:

- Eight glasses of water a day.

- Plenty of fresh fruit and vegetables: Eat at least five portions of fruit and vegetables a day. A single portion is the equivalent of one medium apple, or a palmful of broccoli.

- Plenty of fibre: Choose wholegrain foods such as wholemeal bread, wholegrain cereals, beans, seeds, lentils and other pulses. These help to keep the digestive system functioning well.

- A balanced and varied diet: Choose from a wide variety of healthy foods and vary these each day. Eat fruit and vegetables of lots of different colours, such as orange carrots, dark green spinach, red peppers. This will ensure that you get a wide range of vitamins and minerals. Importantly, don't fall into the trap of eating the same food day in, day out.

- Food that is as fresh as possible: Don't overcook it. Try steaming and grilling instead of deep-frying.

- Plenty of dark green leafy vegetables (such as broccoli and spinach) as these are valuable for strong bones and the avoidance of osteoporosis.

Avoid or restrict your intake of the following:

- alcohol

- caffeine (e.g. coffee, cola)

- foods that are high in sugar, fat or salt, such as fizzy drinks/soda pop, cakes, biscuits/cookies, lollies/sweets/candy, crisps/chips, and fatty deep fried foods (e.g. fish and chips)

- white refined processed foods which are often low in nutritional value but high in sugar, fat and salt (e.g. white bread and pastries)

- ready-made, pre-packaged meals and takeaways that are high in fat and salt and low in nutritional value.

Avoid being overweight. Try to stay within your advised body-weight range. Being overweight places additional strain on your physical structure, which is already working overtime to cope with the asymmetry and imbalance of your scoliosis.

As well as eating good quality food, some people find a few supplements beneficial. For example, Omega-3 fish oils can ease joint inflammation and stiffness. Glucosamine sulphate is often effective in helping to repair stiff, painful and damaged joints, and can be useful for arthritis and back pain. Caution: Consult your doctor before using supplements if you are already on medication, or if you suspect you have a deficiency.

REST

Rest is vital for replenishing the body and enabling it to move and function efficiently. For scoliosis, adequate sleep and rest is particularly important as it restores levels of energy and provides stamina to deal with the imbalance and asymmetry in the physical structure. Without enough sleep, the body becomes fatigued and the twisted scoliotic posture becomes more pronounced as the body slumps and contracts into the helix of the scoliosis.

Try the following:

- Aim for eight hours' sleep each night.

- A siesta or rest for 30–60 minutes during the day (if and when possible) helps to restore stamina and beats fatigue.

- A firm, good quality mattress will support the spine. Avoid beds that sag. A well-sprung quality bed can be very expensive. An alternative way of getting a firm supportive bed is to place a firm board under the mattress (i.e. between the mattress and the base). The board should be the same size as the mattress, and be thick enough not to bend under the weight of your body. A block board 2–3 cm thick is suitable for this purpose.

- Do gentle stretching and flexibility exercises just before going to bed and straight after you rise in the morning. This releases stiffness and tension, and helps keep the spine supple and aligned. (Suitable exercises are described in Part 2.)

- Avoid sleeping on your front or tummy. This puts the spine in an awkward position and places strain on the neck and upper body.

Good sleeping positions

- Lie on your back with a pillow under your knees. This position is kind to the lower back and prevents strain on the lumbar spine.

- Lie on your side with a pillow between your knees. This helps to keep the hips and pelvis aligned.

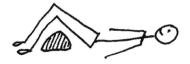 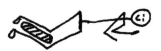

Good sleeping positions

- If you have an unequal waist (with one side straight, and a pronounced curve on the other), lie with the curvy waist side facing down. This helps to encourage the scoliotic spinal curve to flatten out, or at least not to progress. In the event that you do lie with the straight side waist facing down, put a small pad (or rolled-up hand towel) under the waist. This helps prevent the spine from sinking into a deeper curve.

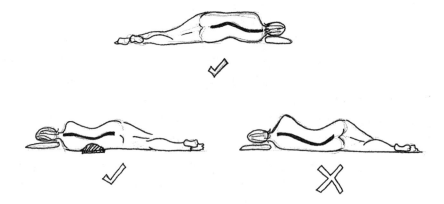

Side lying, curvy waist side down

SITTING

- Don't sit in one position for too long. Get up and stretch every 20–30 minutes if possible.

- In a good sitting position the spine and head are lengthened, and the lower back has a gentle natural lumbar arch. Avoid rounding the spine and slumping forward. This places strain on the back and encourages a twisted scoliotic posture.

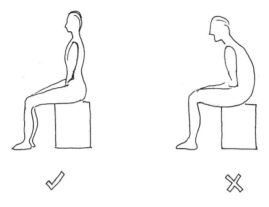

Sitting position

- Check that your weight is placed equally on both buttocks/sit bones. With scoliosis, there is a tendency to shift the weight to one side, usually towards the dominant side with the bossy muscle.

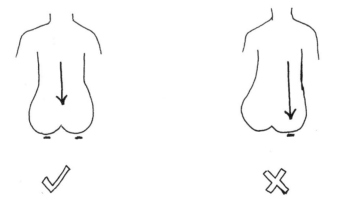

Equal weight distribution when sitting

- Hinge from the hips to lean forward when sitting. This will protect the spine, and maintains the natural lumbar curve and spine length. When working seated at a desk, there is a strong tendency to lean forward towards the computer or book by hunching the head, shoulders and upper body forwards and downwards. This compresses and bends the spine, which leads to aching and stiffness. So, instead of slumping forward, hinge forwards from the hips, keeping your back straight and lengthened.

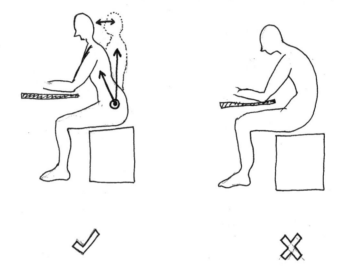

Hinge from the hips

- A good chair is essential. Ideally choose an upright chair which supports your lower back, maintaining the gentle natural curve in the lumbar part of your spine. If necessary, you can make your own lumbar support using a small cushion or a rolled-up towel, or put a lumbar roll behind the small of your back. Here are some ways of modifying a chair to suit your body:

  - If the seat of the chair is too hard, use a flat cushion or a Sissel seat cushion (especially designed for this purpose). This will help avoid compression and stress of the lumbar spine.

  - If the seat is too deep (i.e. your back won't reach the back of the chair), put cushions behind your back for support.

- If the seat is too high (i.e. the soles of your feet can't touch the floor), put cushions under your feet to avoid straining the spine.

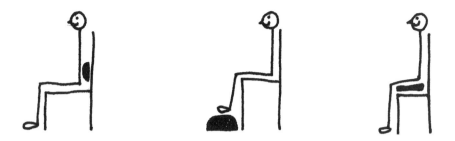

Modifying a chair to suit your body

- Avoid low armchairs and soft sofas. These may look temptingly comfortable, but can hold your back in a compressed rounded position, causing stiffness, bad posture and back pain. If you do have back pain from sofas, there is an alternative way of watching TV that is much kinder to the spine. Lie with your back flat on the floor, with your knees bent and a pillow under your head. It might look a bit antisocial, but it's heaven for your spine!

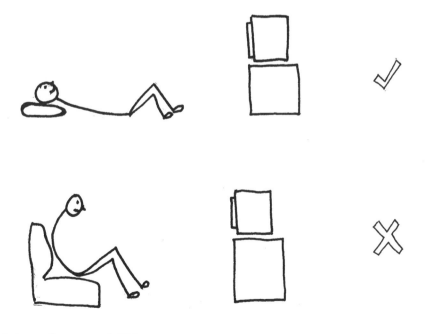

Lying on floor to watch TV

- If your back is aching and stressed while you're sitting, place a tennis ball or spiky massage ball on the aching area and lean backwards onto the back of a chair or a wall. This will give a deep pressure-point massage to the strained area. It also provides additional spine support in sitting position. This technique is particularly good for releasing soreness and tension in the dominant bossy muscles which are strained and overworked from holding a sitting position for too long.

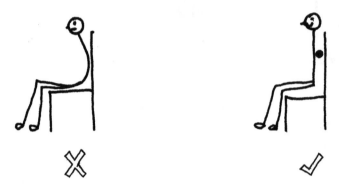

Sitting with ball against the back

- Sitting on the floor, either cross-legged or with legs sideways, can be very uncomfortable and straining for individuals with scoliosis. A good alternative is to sit on a low box or stool (about 15–20 cm high). By raising the bottom off the floor, you can still sit cross-legged, but without the strain and pressure on the spine. Remember to keep a gentle lumbar arch and lengthened head and spine.

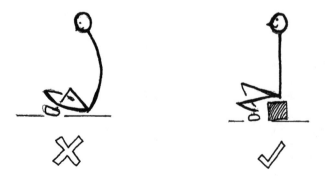

Sitting cross-legged

CARRYING

- Avoid carrying heavy bags.

- Lighten your handbag as much as possible.

- Never use a bag that hangs from your shoulder. This is detrimental for your neck, shoulders and spine. Ideally a small backpack with straps over both shoulders will spread the load evenly.

- Avoid heavy loads, but if you have no choice, divide the load into two bags and hold one in each hand for balance. Do not carry a heavy load on one side only as this creates a severe imbalance and strain on the spine.

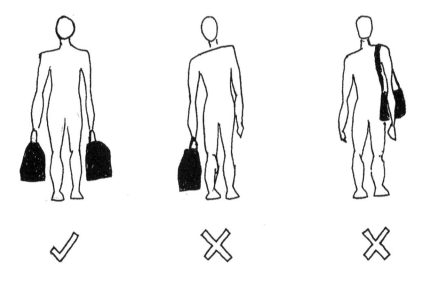

Carrying

STANDING

- In situations where you'll be standing for a long period, wear comfortable supportive shoes.

- Avoid standing still and holding the same position for a long while. For example, if you're waiting in a queue, keep your body flexible and moving:

- ○ Shift the weight onto the balls of your feet, and raise your heels slightly off the ground, and then back down.

- ○ Lift one foot off the ground, and then the other.

- ○ Gently raise and lower your shoulders.

- These movements do not have to be obvious to other people around you. Every few minutes just move your body gently and naturally. Keep your head and spine lengthened and your body relaxed.

- If you're working at a bench (e.g. in the kitchen), check that it is high enough so that you can stand upright with a good comfortable posture. Avoid slouching over the task. Instead, build up the height of the work surface with wooden blocks.

EXERCISE

Physical fitness and exercise are vital for people with scoliosis in keeping the body healthy, strong and flexible. There are two basic types of exercise:

- **Aerobic** or cardiovascular exercise pushes your heart and breathing rate up to supply plenty of oxygen-rich blood to the muscles. This type of exercise gives your heart and lungs a workout and burns off calories. Examples are cycling, swimming and running.

- **Anaerobic** exercise works individual muscles more intensively without increasing the heart rate. Examples of anaerobic exercise are Pilates, yoga and the gentle flexibility exercises described in Part 2.

Both forms of exercise are essential for good health and fitness. Aerobic exercise provides a good cardiovascular workout to the heart and lungs, while anaerobic exercise tones, strengthens and lengthens the muscles and keeps the body supple and flexible.

Because the exercises in this book do not involve a cardiovascular workout, you should supplement your spine flexibility exercises with your choice of aerobic exercise. Try to get a cardiovascular workout at least once a week. Choose whatever you enjoy as long as it doesn't strain or put a negative impact on the spine. Brisk walking, swimming and cycling are ideal aerobic activities.

Avoid high-impact sports where the spine can be jarred and jolted, such as running on hard surfaces without properly sprung shoes. Be careful also of racquet sports and golf, which use one side of the body more than the other. This may further promote the asymmetrical muscle use and imbalance of the scoliosis. Be especially aware if you feel particularly one-sided after playing, or if you sense that the bossy muscle side is overworking.

Gentle forms of non-aerobic exercise include walking, Tai Chi, rehabilitation Pilates and yoga for scoliosis (see Browning Miller 2003). You might find it interesting to explore different ways of using your body in walking (such as that described in *Chi Walking*, by Dreyer and Dreyer 2006).

Summarizing, keep your body moving and fit, and keep your spine flexible, lengthened and strong.

DRESS

Dressing with scoliosis can be seen either as a nightmare or as an opportunity to accept your individuality, think creatively and have some fun. Our bodies with scoliosis are different to the normal figure. Many clothes and designs will simply not suit our particular body shape. This is an opportunity to highlight the good features of your body, and to play down the bits you don't want to focus on. There are some easy and basic tips for covering over and drawing attention away from an unequal torso shape.

Loose fitting clothes

Looser fitting clothes conceal the body shape and are very comfortable. Avoid tight clinging items that accentuate the torso shape. Wear tighter clothes only on the parts of the body that you want to highlight as a good feature. For example, if you've got good legs, and a rib hump, wear a looser fitting top or jacket, and show off your legs with tighter trousers or a skirt.

'Loose fitting' does not mean dressing like a bag lady in shapeless baggy clothes:

- Try garments one size larger for the upper body, if you feel that clothes are unflattering or highlighting bumps that you don't like.

- Try tailored clothes with a sculpted shape that do not cling to the body. For example, a looser jacket with a gently tailored waistline will conceal an unequal waist. Tailored coats left undone create the appearance of an equal waistline.

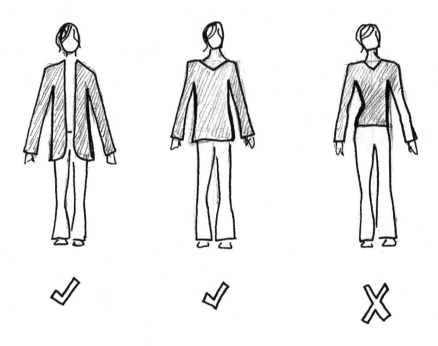

Loose fitting and tailored clothes

Patterned fabric

Small scale prints and fabrics with a patterned texture are an easy and effective way of disguising humps and bumps. Patterned fabric draws attention to the print rather than the body shape underneath.

If you want to wear a tight or clinging garment, try one with a pattern or small scale print. The busyness of the fabric draws the focus away from the asymmetrical body shape.

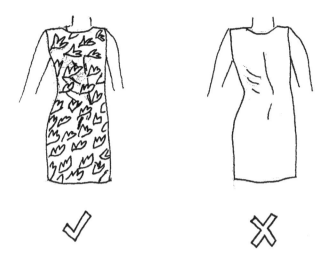

Patterned garments

Darker colours

Darker shades blend in and play down the body shape. Light colours will draw attention to and highlight that part of the body. Avoid the combination of light-coloured, non-patterned, clinging garments because this will highlight every bump and feature.

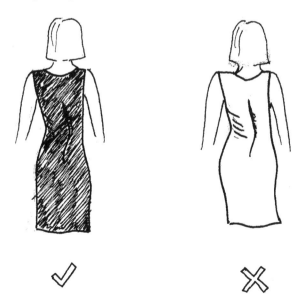

Darker colours conceal

This does not mean that you have to dress in black every day. Black does not suit everyone, and can have a draining washed-out effect. Look for deep tones that suit your complexion. Explore navy blue and indigo, chocolate browns, deep greens, rich burgundy.

There is no rule that says people with scoliosis should always wear dark colours. Simply remember that dark colours disguise the body shape underneath more than light colours do. A tight-fitting, non-patterned garment will look better in a darker colour that disguises the body shape, rather than the same garment in a lighter colour.

Layers

Wearing layers of clothing diverts attention from the shape of the body:

- A loose fitting jacket worn over a T-shirt or polo neck draws attention to the outfit rather than the shape of the body underneath.

- A waist-coat or vest worn unfastened over a loose shirt is versatile and suitable for both casual and more formal occasions.

- An over-shirt worn unbuttoned draws attention away from the shape of the body.

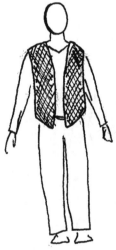
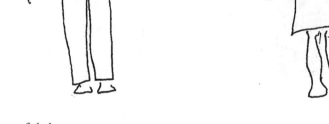

Layers of clothes

Experiment with light, textured, flowing fabrics for outer layer garments. Remember that just a single layer (such as a vest or shirt) worn over a basic garment will disguise any bits that you want to hide.

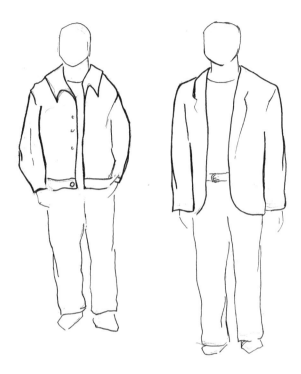

Jacket styles

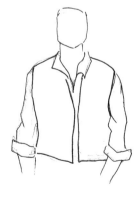

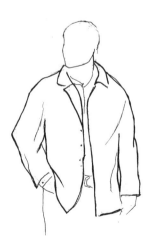

Men's waist-coat   *Overshirt*

Avoid clothes that highlight the waistline

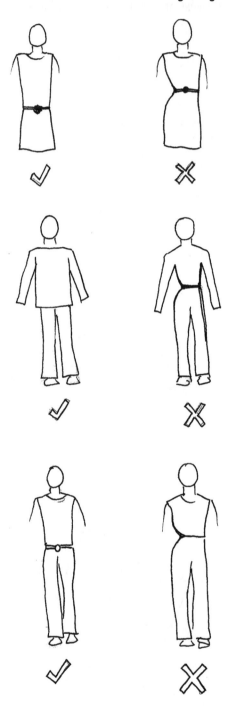

Avoid clothes that highlight the waist

Waistbands and clothes that are belted, gathered or tucked in at the waist are not a good idea if you have an uneven waist. They will only shorten the torso and emphasize the unequal waistline.

Drop-waisted dresses and tops cover up an asymmetrical waist, and create the focus at hip-level instead. Similarly, shirts that are worn outside, rather than tucked in to a waistband, will conceal the waist.

Hipster trousers (i.e. worn on the hips) draw attention away from an uneven waist and also elongate the torso. Avoid high-waisted trousers as this shortens the torso and emphasizes an unequal waistline.

In short, a garment that focuses attention away from the waist, and towards the hips, will disguise an uneven waist and lengthen the torso.

Tailoring

If your job does not allow casual clothes or your lifestyle involves more formal clothing, a lightly tailored jacket in a darker colour worn with a shirt (and tie) works well. Choose a looser jacket rather than a close-fitting one. This will effectively disguise a rib hump and is also more comfortable.

If you have a severe curvature, and your professional life involves wearing suits on a regular basis, you may consider investing in a suit or jacket specifically tailored to suit your individual body shape. If you decide on this option, find the best tailor you can afford who can cut the fabric and construct the shape of the suit to accommodate your particular body form. There are many tricks of the trade that a good tailor will use, such as fitting a foam padding to balance the shape of the body. While this is an expensive option, such a suit will look good for a long time, and can be used as a prototype to copy from in the future at a more reasonable price.

Create focal points

Create focal points with accessories such as jewellery and scarves to divert attention away from the body shape. A plain darker-toned outfit will act as a canvas on which you can create different style statements. This is an opportunity to be creative and have some fun:

- Pieces of jewellery can provide a focal point for an outfit.

- A scarf worn around the neck creates a focus and diverts attention away from the body shape.

- A shawl covers the back and adds interest and style.

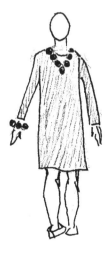 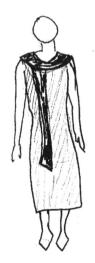 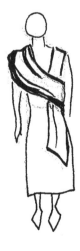

Create focal points

- A sweater or pullover worn casually over the shoulders does a similar job of concealing unequal shoulders and the upper torso.

- Hooded jackets and tops are excellent for covering unequal shoulders, a rib hump and the upper body.

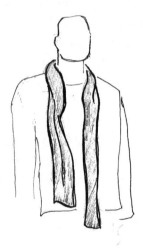

Scarf to create focus

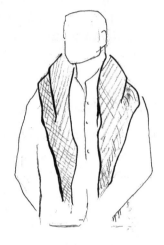

Pullover worn over shoulders

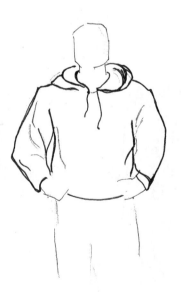

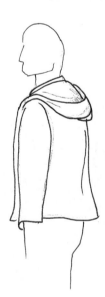

Hooded jacket

Shoes

Invest in a pair of comfortable trainers or flat shoes for everyday casual wear that give good support and are suitable for walking. Where possible, opt for shoes that have flexible softer soles. Hard rigid shoes send shock waves up through your spine as your heels strike the ground. This causes compression and strain on your back. A rigid sole (i.e. one that doesn't bend) restricts the natural flowing movement of your body when walking. This results in bracing and tensing your back to compensate. Trainers are ideal because they are comfortable, flexible and minimize sudden shock waves.

Forget about very high heels and stilettos. They will damage your back and create pain. For smarter, more dressed-up outfits, try heels of 3–5 cm. Avoid higher heels especially if you will be standing or walking for long periods. They throw the spine's natural curves off balance, and thus place stress on the spine and back muscles.

Here are some ideas for how to disguise the following features of scoliosis:

Rib hump:

- layers
- patterned fabric
- darker colours
- shawls and scarves.

Uneven waist:

- drop-waisted and hip-focused garments
- vests and layers
- loose fitting garments that cover the waist.

Uneven shoulders:

- shoulder pad
- scarves
- shawls
- jumper worn over the shoulders

- hooded tops

- long hair.

Unequal hips:

- loose over-garments

- jackets

- to avoid a crooked hemline of skirts and trousers, measure the distance from the hemline to the floor.

For further ideas on dressing with scoliosis, see *Clothes to Suit: Scoliosis and Fashion* by The Scoliosis Association (1994) or *Flatter Your Figure* by Jan Larkey (1992).

HEALTH CARE PLAN

There is no set formula or recipe for dealing with scoliosis. Different things work for different people. It is important to create your own strategies and health care plan for coping with scoliosis, according to your particular condition, preferences and lifestyle.

- First, accept your scoliosis and recognize that it makes you unique. It is a symbol of your individuality.

- Get information about your curvature, so that you understand and are aware of what your scoliosis involves (e.g. location, size and type of the curve(s), the degree of the rib hump).

- Explore the options available for treating your scoliosis and keeping your back strong, lengthened and flexible. Whether or not you have surgery, keep on exploring options and ideas.

- Work out a way forward that best suits you. Look at all of the options and make informed decisions. Make yourself a health care plan for life. Be aware that certain things work well for some people while others find them less effective. Choose the options that you find most effective for you. There is no magic fix, but there are a lot of small measures that when put together make a significant difference, and make living and coping with scoliosis much easier.

As an example, my own health care plan is outlined below. I have made this plan part of my everyday lifestyle and found it effective in keeping my body flexible, healthy and relatively pain-free.

Example of a health care plan

AGE: 50 years

HEIGHT: 5'4"

SPINAL SURGERY: none

CURVATURE: Thoracolumbar curve 60 degrees T10–L5 to right side. Thoracic curve 38 degrees T6–T10 to left side. The curves appear stable. There is no evidence of curve progression.

- Flexibility exercises every day (ten minutes each morning and night).

- Walk at least 30–60 minutes each day.

- Aerobic exercise (e.g. cycling or swimming) once a week.

- Deep tissue massage every one or two weeks.

- Osteopathy when required.

- Eight hours' sleep each night.

- Siesta (one hour's rest) during the day when fatigued.

- Good supportive mattress.

- Healthy and varied diet with plenty of fresh fruit and vegetables.

- Eight glasses of water each day.

- Limited intake of alcohol and caffeine.

- Avoid junk food and processed foods high in sugar, fat and salt.

- Avoid excess body weight.

- Select a good chair.

- Frequent stretch breaks with desk work.

- Keep moving – don't sit or stand in one position for too long. Move and stretch every 20 minutes if possible.

- Avoid carrying heavy loads. Lighten your handbag.

- Wear comfortable and supportive shoes, especially for standing and walking.

- Be aware of your posture when sitting and standing. Keep the spine lengthened and the head floating upwards. Make sure your weight is equally balanced between left and right sides of the body.

- Buy a vehicle with heated seats, good suspension and neck support, if possible.

If the pain gets bad:

- Heated back pad (e.g. Thermacare pain relieving heatwrap).

- Hot bath in Radox.

- Lie on the floor with knees bent, and two pillows under the knees.

- Gentle flexibility exercises if and when possible.

CASE STUDIES

Scoliosis encompasses enormous variation and each person's scoliosis is different. The case studies below are stories of some individuals with different degrees of curvature, experiences and ways of coping. (For privacy, all names have been changed.)

A L I

AGE: 15 years

CURVATURE: Thoracic curve (approximately 30 degrees) to the right.
                Kyphosis (forward bending of the upper back).

SURGERY: None

I've got a minor curve leaning to the right side which is noticeable as a 'hump' if I bend over. The curve is around the centre section of my back and causes a lot of pain.

I was 13, nearly 14, when my mother noticed a small 'hump' slightly to the right of the centre of my back. Later, this was diagnosed as scoliosis. This was only minor but it prevented me from practising heavy activities easily such as major weightlifting and rugby. This was a relief, as it could have been worse.

Several doctors saw my back and said not to do any heavy lifting. I had an MRI (Magnetic Resonance Imaging) scan which showed a small piece in my spinal cord had fused wrong. I still get pains from time to time if I stand up too long or lift too many heavy objects. Not many people know the full extent of my back problem because I cope with it and wear loose clothing. This prevents me from getting hassle. It won't get worse unless I overstrain myself.

I find Alexander technique lessons help. Also I try to work out at least once or twice a week. I do Karate once a week which gives me confidence and control. If I'm working at the computer, it's important to take a break and stretch out. If I'm sore from standing for too long, I sit down and stretch occasionally. It's important not to over-stretch though. I wear slightly looser clothes than normal, and avoid wearing jeans with a tight waist, especially if I'm going to work out.

Marion's story (Ali's mother)

Ali spends too much time on the computer – like many teenage boys! One day while he was crouched over some medieval war game I noticed a rather strange hump on the right-hand side of his spine. I thought it must be his position at the computer – or a muscle abnormality because he was spending too much time online. I ignored it and hoped it would go away. But then several months later when he was bending over getting something out of his school bag I noticed the 'hump' was even more pronounced.

When he stood up straight, it vanished. I could feel nothing unusual on that side of his back. But then I remembered a 'forward-bend' test that we had to do at the beginning of each term at school. A friend I'd hung around with in my teens had discovered a curvature of her spine which had turned out to be serious. She was operated on and, for what seemed like months afterwards, she was incarcerated in a full body plaster. Several of us were drafted in to carry her school bags for a time. She coped very cheerfully, but it can't have been much fun at that stage of life when we were all obsessing over our bodies. I imagined Ali in a full body plaster, me putting on his socks and carrying his bag…

I thought the doctor would dismiss my fears.

But she didn't. She sent us off to the spine specialist. Ali had X-rays, then MRI imaging. Yes, there was a curvature. And several fused ribs. He pored over the X-rays and images. Ali had probably been born this way, but it had only become apparent in adolescence. We were sent to the head honcho at a large hospital. We were reassured that he'd seen many worse cases. Ali's really wasn't that interesting. Not interesting enough to operate anyway. But they'd see us every six months to keep an eye on things.

They thought he'd almost stopped growing so things were not likely to get much worse.

Sometimes though it's easy to fear the worst and I found it reassuring to talk with different people about various options and ways of coping.

My husband had a slight 'kink' in his spine in the 1980s which he had treated successfully with the Alexander technique so we arranged to see an Alexander teacher who was recommended to us. Ali immediately liked him and now sees him once a month or so. He's taught Ali how to 'release' his back and to relax. Ali enjoys being inches higher after his Alexander lessons and he certainly seems more relaxed.

We are due back at the specialist next month and we'll see how things have developed. Ali is learning to live with his kyphoscoliosis and to manage the pain – and we've had great support on the journey.

SAMANTHA

AGE: 42 years

CURVATURE: Before surgery, an S-shape curve: thoracic curve (T6–T11) 48 degrees to the right. Lumbar curve (T11–L4) 50 degrees to the left.

SURGERY: Harrington rods and spinal fusion T6–T11 at age 13. Minimal thoracic curve after operation. Lumbar curve remains.

My scoliosis was first noticed when I was about 12. I was in a dress shop trying on a strapless dress when the woman in the shop exclaimed 'Wow, either my dressmaking is out or your daughter's hip is out!' My mum took me to see our local doctor, who then referred me to a specialist.

For six months I was doing daily exercises tailored to try and prevent further curvature of the spine, with no aim of surgery.

After six months my scoliosis had progressed dramatically and so I was then referred to another specialist in the city. We all liked him a lot. He explained things really clearly, using models and drawings. He showed me a model of my spine and explained what was happening to it. He said that the degree of curvature was now too severe to be rectified by exercise or bracing alone and, as I still had another two years of bone growth to go, surgery was recommended. I remember walking into the lift with my dad and bursting into tears!

So at 13 I flew back to the city with my mum and my sister for the surgery. On the morning of the operation, I thought 'This is the last shower I will ever have without Harrington rods fused to my spine'. My nerves washed away when they were prepping me for surgery. Mum was putting on a brave face. Next thing I was being taken to theatre, now that was another world! When I woke up, Mum was crying and I told her to stop. I realized then that the operation was complete.

The operation was a short thoracic fusion using metal rods, screws and hooks at either end, causing this section of my spine to straighten, correcting my rib hump. Bone chips were taken from my hip and spine and packed around the rods to help it knit and fuse my spine. That section of my spine is now solid and stable and cannot bend or grow (at the time I had two years to go before I reached skeletal maturity). However, the lumbar curve was left as is and has movement with no fusion. My operation took over five hours. There was no rib removal.

While I was in intensive care I sucked on ice first. Then I was moved to a ward where I could have food (including sweet strawberries – you couldn't get those in my home town!). All in all I was in hospital for seven weeks lying on my back with a mirror mounted above me so that I could see people who came to visit. I was fitted with a body cast to support my spine during recovery. After several weeks lying down I had to learn to walk again.

I got home to a new waterbed. After three months of really hot weather I went back to the city for a check-up where they cut off the plaster cast. I thought 'Wow, my skin can breathe'. Then they put on a new one and I flew back home with Mum.

After seven months my body cast was removed. I felt like a turtle without its shell and my neck looked too long (the shoulders on the plaster cast were a lot higher than my own). It was nice to be able to eat dinner without my belly sticking out of the hole they'd cut in the cast, and to get rid of the chewing gum that some kid had thrown down the back of my cast during class.

Scoliosis is definitely hereditary in my family. My grandmother, mother and sister also have it. While we were at the children's hospital for my operation, the specialist checked my younger sister's back and found her to be clear of scoliosis. Six months later, she too had scoliosis and ended up having surgery; it all happened that fast!

Spinal surgery techniques constantly improve and advance at a fast rate. My sister didn't have to wear a plaster cast for the last three months like I did. Instead she had a brace which she could unclip in the shower. (We called her 'Ned' because she looked like Ned Kelly, the Australian bushranger!)

I'm glad I've had surgery because if I didn't then my life would be very different to what it is now. You can barely see my scar and only three people have ever asked me about it. Once was when I was 18 and set off the metal detector at the airport, so I just showed them my scar.

I went back to see the surgeon for a check-up about 12 years ago. It was good to see him again and to know that he's still practising. He thought that my back was fine and said that when people have surgery these days, they're up and walking in a few days. Surgical techniques have improved and they now fix the rods to each vertebra, rather than at the top and bottom of the curve like they did with mine.

My husband and I now share our lives with our son. I had a dream pregnancy and enjoyed the experience of labour. I ended up having to have an emergency Caesarean and I think that was purely because I've still got a lumbar curve (which wasn't fused).

I've never had any problems because of the operation. The key to that is exercise and good well-being. I keep active and enjoy walking along the beach with my husband and son and our dogs, and sometimes swimming.

LOUISE

AGE: 55 years

CURVATURE: Thoracic curve 60 degrees to the right. Compensatory cervical and lumbar curves to the left.

SURGERY: Spinal fusion and rods inserted T6–T10. Two ribs removed.

My scoliosis was first noticed when I was 13. When I was home for the Easter holidays from boarding school, my grandfather spotted it, commenting that my right shoulder was higher than the left. At first they thought it might be polio. When we went to the doctor, he had X-rays done and diagnosed scoliosis. The orthopaedic specialist told me the curve was progressing rapidly and that I needed an operation or could end up in a wheelchair. For the next year we saw many specialists and tried different treatments. I was doing physiotherapy, swimming, weights and back strengthening exercises. They even put me on a rack for 20 minutes at a time to stretch out my spine.

By the time I was 15, it was obvious my back was getting worse and so I decided to go ahead with the operation. They fused T6–T10 and cut out the two bottom ribs, ground them up and packed them around the spine. For three months afterwards I had to wear a big structured back brace with two outside rods, taking it off only in bed at night. About five months after the operation, I was on a ride at a fun fair and jolted my spine. I remember that massive pain. I discovered afterwards that the bottom screw on my spine had snapped in two. When I went back to the specialist a couple of years later, he said that in retrospect he could have fused more, from T5 to T11, because it would have made me straighter.

I was very self-conscious of my back. I felt like I was deformed. One breast was larger than the other, my ribs were crooked and I was very aware of the hump around my right shoulder blade area. As a teenager I was really protective of my back and hesitated and held back from letting boys close to me.

I found the operation and the recuperation traumatic. However, after all of that was over, all in all my back was good. I got on with my life. In my 20s and 30s I had a really active life doing everything, travelling, hiking, sailing, dancing and all with no pain.

In my early 40s, all of that changed. I started getting back pain when I took a job that involved driving over rough corrugated roads, constantly bumping and jolting up and down. Then one day the truck hit a large pothole in the road and from then on I had major problems.

Since then I've had a limited life with lots of pain. The pain is always there and now 12 years down the track it's dismaying. It affects me psychologically. I feel distressed and suffer depression as a result of the chronic pain. If I'm stressed the pain is worse. The more the stress, the worse the pain. Then the pain creates more stress and so the vicious cycle continues. I now feel very self-conscious about my body. I'm hesitant to show anyone my body. I don't go swimming in public places and always wear baggy clothes to cover up and disguise it.

A neurosurgeon says that my spine is more degenerated than that of an 80-year-old, but I try to keep as active as I can and refuse to be a victim. I am now limited to gentle movement and very light physical activity like slow walking and gentle lengthening and stretching exercises. No carrying heavy loads or sitting or standing in one position for long. Sweeping and hoovering create pain. I can no longer work but can do light chores around the house and move around gently. I need lots of rest each day as I feel constantly exhausted. I do what I can, try to keep positive and look on the bright side.

Scoliosis has changed my life big time. You become a different person. It's made me an individual.

P H O E B E

AGE: 36 years

CURVATURE: Lumbar curve approximately 30 degrees to the left (L1–L5), with a small compensatory thoracic curve to the right.

SURGERY: None

As long as I can remember I've had scoliosis. It was something I grew up with. My mother has the same condition. During my childhood and teenage years, my parents searched for different ways to treat my spinal curve. When I was 14, we went to an orthopaedic surgeon who took X-rays and measurements of my back. It showed that the main curvature is in my lower back [a lumbar curve of 30 degrees leaning to the left]. The consultant advised us that nothing could be done. It was not worth having surgery because the curve was too small. We thus realized that the operation was not an option for me.

I really don't remember scoliosis affecting me very much as a teenager. I kept very active doing sports like windsurfing, mountain biking and horse riding. At college, work and uni, friends would sometimes tease me about sitting on a cushion but apart from that it was OK.

At the start of my 20s, I became more aware of my scoliosis. I felt that my body was getting shorter. My shortened torso seemed to make me look overweight and I became conscious of my weight and body shape. When I was 26, I really started focusing on my fitness, going to the gym, Nordic walking, swimming, cycling and horse riding. Doing all this now, I keep as active as possible.

There are a few challenges. It's difficult to buy clothes because of my short torso and one hip being higher than the other. Clinging material and tight outfits show my body and highlight my unequal hips so I've learnt to avoid them. Instead I wear hip-length tops and coats to cover my torso. Flat shoes are best to avoid back pain.

Pain is the other challenge. If I sit or stand for too long my back gets really sore now. Sitting on hard surfaces is especially painful so I always carry a cushion. Some activities like running, hoovering and carrying heavy loads create a lot of discomfort so I avoid doing them.

What works best for me physically is keeping healthy and fit. I keep active and I keep on moving as much as possible. I do lots of sport and have regular one-on-one Pilates sessions for flexibility and posture. Massage and physiotherapy treatments are very helpful for releasing tight muscle areas and discomfort in my back. There are some basic lifestyle tips that I follow to stay as healthy as possible with my curvature. A lot of sleep and rest is essential. I have a good mattress. I eat a healthy diet and try to keep the weight off. The more weight I lose, the better my back is. Stretching and gentle exercises keep my back flexible. I avoid sitting or standing for long periods. I walk wearing flat shoes, and try to avoid hard surfaces because this jolts my spine.

My way of coping is to keep moving and stay active. I don't get embarrassed about using cushions and props, and don't worry about what people think. I just enjoy life.

THERESA

AGE: 45 years

CURVATURE: Thoracolumbar curve 45 degrees to the right.

SURGERY: Spinal fusion and rods inserted T4–L2, at age 11.

When I was four years old, the doctor noticed that I had curvature of the spine. In those days the treatment for scoliosis was to lie on a hard gypsum bed, strapped in so you couldn't move. I had to do this every night for two years. I remember crying all night and feeling unloved and distressed. After that, the next treatment was a corset, but I refused to wear it at school because I felt so ashamed.

When I was 13, the doctor suggested surgery for my spine. I agreed to the operation. Because I had a large curve [65 degrees] that could progress, I felt I had no choice. The surgery inserted two rods in my thoracic spine fusing 11 vertebrae from T4 to L2. This reduced my curve from 65 degrees to 24 degrees. This form of operation was new in 1976. There was little knowledge of how spinal fusion would affect the vertebrae above and below the rigid fused section of the spine. [Since this time, surgery has greatly improved and is now much advanced.]

For three months after the operation, my body was encased in a big corset like a cast. I was not allowed to sit and had to kneel on the floor to eat at the table. Three months later I was given a new corset and was then able to sit down on a chair.

As a young person, I was traumatized by this corset. It was like being in prison. I was totally dependent on other people for going to the toilet. I had no privacy. It was torture for my body. The corset was big and bulky and it was so high that it wore the hair away on the back of my head. After the removal of the corset, at a disco I was nicknamed 'hamster' because the corset had touched my face and pushed my cheeks upwards.

In my 20s I worked as a dental assistant. The constant bending over and leaning forward gave me a lot of back pain and headaches, so eventually I gave up that work. The fused section of my back is OK, but the areas above and below the fused section are very painful. Now in my 40s, I'm experiencing more pain and am aware of my spine becoming rigid. I don't know how much longer I'll be able to cut my toenails because of my spine stiffening.

My curve has now increased to 45 degrees and I have a rib hump. Clothes are a problem. I can't often find clothes that fit and can't wear many styles. Sometimes I feel embarrassed about my body.

I like to stay positive although there are quite a few things I avoid doing now like tennis, horse riding, jumping and carrying heavy loads. I don't sit down for long in one place and don't sweep because it causes me pain. Sometimes my hands feel paralysed. The best things for me are gentle light exercise, massage and heat treatments.

I cope by living one day at a time and not worrying about the past or the future. There are people who are worse off than me. I look at all of the good things in life and have great faith in my Creator God and optimism.

ISOBEL

AGE: 15 years

CURVATURE: Thoracolumbar curve (28 degrees) to the left side (T12–L4).

SURGERY: None

My curvature of the spine was first noticed when I was eight years old. I'd just had the first operation for my pacemaker and my back started to get really sore. My mum took me to a physiotherapist and she asked us to bring along the X-ray of my pacemaker (because you can see my spine in it). It was then discovered that I had a slight curve of around 20 degrees.

I didn't get upset or worried when we were told that I had scoliosis. I was just a child, eight years old, and I didn't really understand. At that time my heart arrhythmia and getting through pacemaker operations were the most urgent and important things, and that's what we focused on.

When I was 11 years old, I had a second operation to have the pacemaker replaced and the wires in my heart positioned properly. Whilst in the children's hospital there, they gave me a really thorough health check and the doctor advised us to get an appointment with an orthopaedic specialist to check on my spine.

My first check-up with the orthopaedic surgeon was tense and I didn't really like it. I was very young and felt uncomfortable. Unfortunately he could offer no solution to my back pain which I desperately wanted. He said 'lots of people suffer back pain' and that scoliosis does not cause back pain or something to that effect. I remember being very upset when I left the surgery and didn't want to go back for any more appointments.

Since then I have had my back checked every six months by another orthopaedic specialist closer to home, who monitors my degree of curvature. Last year the check-up showed that the curvature had progressed from 22 degrees to 28 degrees. We became very worried that the curve might keep on increasing. Fortunately the latest check-up appointment indicated that my curvature seems to have stabilized again. It hasn't moved past 28 degrees and that's encouraging.

We've decided to wait and watch and monitor the curve closely. We'll see what the next appointment brings. I'm now back seeing the original orthopaedic surgeon. (I don't mind seeing him now – as I'm older and more confident.) At the last appointment he said that surgery is an option but not an urgent priority, unless the scoliosis is causing me great concern cosmetically.

The very mention of surgery or even wearing a brace made me fearful when I was younger. My view has changed as I've got older and now I'd perhaps consider surgery so that my spine could be straight again.

Having scoliosis hasn't really impacted that much on my lifestyle. I don't have intense pain like I used to, so that makes it easier to put up with. I still get some pain when I'm sitting studying for long periods or standing in one spot for a long time. Heat pads, stretching out my spine, and changing sitting and standing position are good ways for me to relieve tension and discomfort in my back.

One side of my back is thicker than the other. I don't like it but it's not that bad. I wear loose clothes and T-shirts so people can't see my back.

My heart condition and operations at an early age put life in perspective for me. I don't really worry all that much about my curvature of the spine. I feel that there are other people with much bigger curvatures, and people much worse off than me. I stay calm and centred and just live life to the full.

EMILY

AGE: 40 years

CURVATURE: Thoracic curve to the right side.

SURGERY: Harrington rod and spinal fusion at age 12.

The operation for my scoliosis was in October 1981. I was 12 years old. The post-operation period was not difficult for me as my sister had been through it all, and I knew what to expect. I had been with her to all her check-ups. The only thing I hated about the whole hospital experience was when the young doctor students came to my room by the dozen and the doctors removed my sheets to show my back! I felt very intimidated.

Apart from that, the three weeks I spent lying on my back in hospital went very quickly. The nurses were very friendly, joyful and playful. They were always making sure we had something to do from the art trolley. Sometimes some of the other sick children would come in and visit me. The biggest experience was when they decided it was time to wash my hair! They slid me up to the top of the bed, tilted the bed up so my head was lowest and my legs and body were up in the air! I felt like a human slippery dip [playground slide] and that I was going to slide out. We had a big laugh about it!

Luckily I had Mum's support through the whole experience. She had to catch a bus to and from the hospital every day to visit. I don't know what I would have done without her. It can't have been easy going through the same procedure twice in a short time. She was always positive and I don't remember being negative.

I remember feeling proud after having the operation, just like I was so brave and I'd managed some big achievement in my life. I wasn't very popular in school, so it felt good to have a bit of attention!

Later when we joined the swimming club, I didn't mind people noticing my scar to be honest. It never bothered me. I felt proud and had no problems explaining about it when people asked. I'd tell them: 'After the operation I am 2 cm longer and I had 153 stitches, 150 dissolving ones and 3 normal ones!'

Although I was never really good with contact sports, I found other sports that suited me. I always loved my swimming and, when we moved 5 kilometres out of town, I used to ride my bike to and from school. Then I started canoeing and I entered in several Red Cross canoed marathons (86 km race over two days). I also did a quadrathon, where I paddled 13 km, and then jogged 5 km. In all of which I raised money for the Red Cross. It was a lot of fun.

At the age of 20 I moved to Europe to be with my boyfriend. That was 20 years ago and we are still going strong! My sporting activities have toned down to an exercise bike during the winter, as well as Pilates and swimming a kilometre every day during summer.

Now, my scar is not really noticeable. Nobody asks me about it and my hair is quite long, so it's probably covering what little scar there is left. I've been to a few doctors in Europe, just for check-ups. All of them have said that the specialist did a really good job with my back operation. I have had no complications whatsoever.

All I can say is that I'm happy for having the operation. Our local doctor explained everything to us so clearly and I had no doubt that the operation was best for me. The surgeon did a very good job, but it is the after-process that is just as important.

You have to change your life according to it and try your best to keep some sort of routine. It is my willpower, devotion, a basic interest in eating right and regular exercises that is my success story. That is why at 40 my body looks better than that of most 25-year-olds. I am especially proud that it does as I have scoliosis.

I do Pilates exercises every day. Swimming and cycling are fantastic! I try to keep my weight constant and don't let it get out of control. I am 165 cm tall and have weighed between 52 and 55 kilos for the past 20 years. Don't let your scoliosis be an excuse not to take care of yourself. Tell yourself you need to take care of your back and you will feel confident, healthy and happy for doing so.

GLOSSARY

Adductors: Inner thigh muscles.

Aerobic exercise: Exercise that raises the heart rate and makes you breathe harder to deliver more oxygen to the muscles, e.g. swimming, cycling, very brisk walking.

Asymmetrical: With one side unequal to the other. In contrast, 'symmetrical' means equal and balanced on both sides.

Cervical spine: Begins at the base of the skull and includes the neck area.

Cobb angle: System for measuring the degree or angle of a spine curved with scoliosis.

Concave: The open mouth side of a curve.

Convex: The side which a curve leans towards (i.e. the outside of the curve).

Core stability: By strengthening the muscles in the centre of the body, you can keep the pelvis and spine in correct alignment. Core stability is one of the key goals of general Pilates.

Disc: Fibrous disc-shaped cartilage between the vertebrae of the spine, acting as a shock absorber.

Engaging the abdominals: Pulling the stomach muscles in toward the back.

Extension: If you are asked to extend an arm or a leg in an exercise, it means you straighten it.

Facet joints: The small joints at the back of the spine that link the vertebrae together. There are two facet joints between each pair of vertebrae, one on each side. Facet joints are vital in keeping the entire spinal column stable yet flexible.

Flat back: Excessive flattening of the back so that the spine (viewed sideways) loses its gentle natural curve.

Flexion: Flexion generally means bending. If you are asked to flex your elbow, you bend it.

Glutes or **gluteus maximus muscles:** These are the buttock muscles. They help straighten the hip and rotate the hip joint outward.

Hamstrings: Muscles down the backs of the thighs that help bend the knee and straighten the hip. It is important to stretch these muscles, because tight hamstrings cause the pelvis to tip out of alignment.

Hip flexors: Group of muscles in the hip region that allow you to lift your knee and bend at the waist.

Idiopathic: Simply means that the cause is unknown.

Kyphoscoliosis: Combination of scoliosis (sideways curvature of the spine) and kyphosis (forward bending of the upper back).

Kyphosis: Pronounced forward curve of the upper back.

Lateral: To the side. Lateral bending means bending to one side.

Lordosis: Pronounced arching of the lower back, causing the stomach and bottom to stick out.

Lumbar: Lower back. The lumbar spine is that part of the spine below the waist.

Pelvic alignment: The pelvis is able to tilt backwards and forwards (as in 'Pelvic rocks', exercise 9). However, for daily movements and activities, it should be held by the surrounding muscles in an alignment that doesn't put any strain on the spine. If you have a lumbar scoliosis with one hip pushed further forward or higher than the other, it is important to focus on gently realigning your pelvis. Note that pelvic alignment may be thrown out of balance if you frequently sit with your legs crossed, or if you wear high heels.

Pelvic floor: The hammock of muscles between the legs. Keeping these muscles strong can prevent incontinence in later life.

Physio ball: A large rubber ball used in Pilates and physiotherapy exercises.

Psoas: A major muscle connecting the lower spine, pelvic area and hip joint. It is responsible for stabilizing the base of the spine, hip movement, and allowing the spine to flex.

Quads or **quadriceps:** Muscles at the front of the thigh, which enable you to straighten the leg and raise the thigh.

Rib hump: A prominence or bulge on one side of the back, caused by the rib cage twisting to one side.

Rotation: Turning around a central axis. With scoliosis, rotated vertebrae turn around the vertical axis of the spine, like stairs in a spiral staircase.

Stenosis: Narrowing of the spaces in the spine resulting in compression of the nerve roots or spinal cord.

Thoracic: The thoracic spine extends from the upper back between the shoulders down to the waist. (Thorax is the medical name for chest.)

Thoracolumbar: Affecting both the thoracic (upper back down to the waist) and lumbar (lower back) areas of the spine.

Vertebrae: Individual bones of the spine. Vertebrae are stacked on top of each other from the tailbone to the base of the skull to form the spinal column. The adult spine has approximately 33 vertebrae, including five that are fused to form the sacrum, and four which are fused to form the tailbone.

REFERENCES

Browning Miller, E. (2003) *Yoga for Scoliosis*. Palo Alto, California: Shanti Productions, LLC.

Dreyer, D. and Dreyer, K. (2006) *Chi Walking: The Five Mindful Steps for Lifelong Health and Energy*. New York: Simon & Schuster.

Hawes, M.C. (2003) *Scoliosis and the Human Spine: A Critical Review of Clinical Approaches to the Treatment of Spinal Deformity in the United States, and a Proposal for Change*. Tucson, Arizona: West Press.

Larkey, J. (1992) *Flatter Your Figure*. New York: Simon & Schuster.

Lehnert-Schroth, C. (2007) *Three-Dimensional Treatment for Scoliosis: A Physiotherapeutic Method for Deformities of the Spine*. Palo Alto, California: The Martindale Press.

Schommer, N. (2002) *Stopping Scoliosis: The Whole Family Guide to Diagnosis and Treatment*. New York: Avery (Penguin Putnam).

Selby, A. and Herdman, A. (1999) *Pilates: Creating the Body You Want*. London: Gaia Books.

The Scoliosis Association (UK) (1994) *Clothes to Suit: Scoliosis and Fashion*. London: SAUK.

Weiss, R.H. (2006) *'Best Practice' in Conservative Scoliosis Care*. Munich: Richard Pflaum Verlag.

ABOUT THE AUTHORS

ANNETTE WELLINGS

Annette Wellings is a trained Pilates instructor. As a person with major scoliosis, she has explored different ideas, strategies and exercises for coping with scoliosis in everyday living. This book is the result.

Annette was born in tropical Australia. She worked as a linguist in Japanese, Australian Aboriginal languages and Fijian and has lived extensively in these cultures. She also worked for some years as a textile designer and artist in Australia.

While following a career as a linguist and an artist, Annette became increasingly aware of her body becoming more hunched and painful with scoliosis. She began exploring different options and ways of keeping the body flexible and healthy with scoliosis. Consequently she trained in rehabilitation Pilates, studying in London with Alan Herdman. This book describes some ideas, strategies and exercises that she has found effective in coping with scoliosis in adulthood.

ALAN HERDMAN

Alan Herdman is the leading practitioner of the Pilates technique in the UK. Having learnt the method in New York, he introduced Pilates to the UK in 1970, and has established exercise studios there and in several other countries. Alan is also a Laban-trained teacher of Dance Drama and he studied the Graham Technique at the London School of Contemporary Dance.

He continues to adapt and develop new exercises to address the need of every client he consults with. He teaches doctors, professional dancers, actors, sportsmen and women, and all kinds of people with a huge variety of physical problems. His first book, *Pilates: Creating the Body You Want* (Selby and Herdman 1999), is a worldwide best-seller.

INDEX